YOGA
TAICHI
REIKI

A GUIDE FOR ALL CHRISTIANS

Max Sculley DSL

Modotti Press
AN IMPRINT OF CONNOR COURT PUBLISHING

Connor Court Publishing Pty Ltd.
PO Box 1
Ballan VIC 3342
sales@connorcourt.com
www.connorcourt.com

ISBN: 9781921421716 (pbk.)

Cover design by Ian James

Printed in Australia

CONTENTS

Foreword by Bishop Julian Porteous   1

Preface   7

PART A: YOGA

1. Out of India   13
2. The Philosophy of Yoga   29
3. From the Holy Spirit?   41
4. Monkeying with Minds in the Monastery   53
5. A Genuine Christian Alternative to Yoga   69

PART B: TAI CHI

6. Just an Innocent Pastime   73
7. Taoist Philosophy   91
8. To Chi or not to Chi   99

PART C: REIKI

9. A Crypto-Religion   111
10. Reiki Wreckage   127
11. Rating Reiki   141

PART D: THE AGE OF AQUARIUS

12. New Age Fallacies   151

Endnotes   155

Glossary   167

I consecrate this book through the

Immaculate Heart of Mary to the

All Merciful Heart of Jesus.

Acknowledgements

To those confreres and friends who have supported and encouraged me in the writing of the book, a special thank you.

To my local community of De La Salle Brothers who have generously funded the publication of the book, a special thanks. I hasten to add that this fraternal support does not imply agreement with the views expressed here for which the author takes sole responsibility.

To my group of editorial advisers who patiently read over successive editions of the manuscript and gave me valuable feedback: Brother Fabian Clarke fsc (recently deceased) who had a great ability to go quickly to the heart of things and who was possessed of a special gift of discernment of spirits; Susie Bennett for her wisdom and attention to detail; Diane Wood whose past experience in New Age and wise guidance has proved invaluable; Steve Bennett for his support and business acumen.

To all those who allowed me to interview them and who provided their testimonies for publication I am most grateful. For reasons of confidentiality, names of persons and places have been altered in all testimonies.

To Eric Harz and his publisher Jubilee Resources for permission to use extensive material from his book *The Reiki Danger: Healing that Harms* a special thanks for giving me an excellent introduction to the Reiki culture.

To Tony Anthony for permission to use extensive material from his fascinating book *Taming the Tiger*, a special thanks for giving me such valuable insights into the nature of tai chi underpinning Kung Fu.

To Aaron Turnbull, Managing Director of Turnbull Marketing & Design, I thank you and your staff members for your patience, flexibility and competence in producing all the graphic design work.

To Kevin Tan, thanks for your fine art work, only some of which appears in the present volume.

To Sue Crouch, thank you for your patience and demanding work in typing the final version and also for encouraging me to complete the work.

To Alan McDermott, thank you for your speedy and professional printing of the final stages of the manuscript, often going well beyond the call of duty.

And a big thank you to Bishops Julian Porteous and Peter Elliott for your encouragement to publish the book and for endorsing it upon publication.

Finally, with a glance into the past, thank you to the staff of the now-defunct Institute of Formative Spirituality (Duquesne University Pittsburgh) who helped me develop my critical and discerning faculties.

Unless otherwise indicated, all scriptural quotations are from *The New Jerusalem Bible.*

Foreword

Yoga, Tai Chi, Reiki are now familiar terms to most Australians. While these practices and the accompanying philosophies have been introduced to Australia in relatively recent times, they have been accepted quite readily by many people. Indeed, they have become very popular. Almost every suburb or country town would provide access to these practices and techniques which are seen as means to relaxation. Many people have not only made use of the practices, but have gone on to learn how to teach the techniques. Many have submitted themselves to a more detailed exploration of the spiritual background to the practices. Many have oriented their lives around the philosophies that underpin these techniques. The experiences associated with the use of the techniques have opened up doors into a new spiritual world, the world of Eastern religions.

As techniques they have been marketed as good for relaxation, fitness and general health. They are now widely used with this purpose in mind. Most would view them as being beneficial at the physical and emotional levels. These techniques are seen as a source of personal wellbeing. Few would question whether there are any dangerous aspects to these practices.

Devotees of these techniques would claim that they do not have a religious dimension. They would claim that anyone can keep their own beliefs and utilise these practices for the good they offer. They are viewed as useful techniques that anyone of any or no religious background can utilise.

On the understanding that they are not religious but are merely techniques, they have been successfully integrated into mainstream Australian life. Sports people use them. Business people turn to them. Many Christians have been drawn to them, seeing them as supplementing Christian spiritual practices.

This book, *Yoga, Tai Chi & Reiki*, by Br Max Sculley, provides an invaluable insight into the background to these practices. His research reveals the underlying 'philosophies' or world views that have given rise to these techniques. He shows clearly that using the techniques leads many into a new spiritual world. These practices and techniques cannot be viewed as only being of benefit at the physical and emotional levels. Of their very nature they draw a person into the spiritual realm. The techniques rely not only on physical movement but engage a person in entering into an altered state of consciousness. Their powers derive from engagement with the spiritual world. Persons utilising the practices will be invited to engage their minds with the techniques in order for them to have any real benefit. This is where the danger lies.

This world into which the practitioner is introduced is inimical to the Christian faith. While they may offer practices that can be helpful at a superficial level they are a Trojan horse for dangerous spiritual infiltration. In their desire to know more of the technique which they have found beneficial a person can unwittingly be exposed to demonic powers. They have ventured into a mysterious world lacking the sound guidance that Christianity offers. When one encounters preternatural powers the question does need to be posed: what is the origin and nature of these powers? If they are not from the God revealed by Jesus Christ, then where do they come from? Venturing further into this exotic world can lead a person to embracing a belief in and a personal subjection to powers that do not come from the true God. Indeed, a person who follows these religious philosophies to their full extent can find themselves worshipping a false God.

There are a number of common elements to Yoga, Tai Chi and

Reiki. They all offer a physical practice that is readily accessible. They claim to offer methods that achieve relaxation and offer paths to greater wellbeing and healing. Many people find this to be the case. At the superficial level of these systems there may be no more than the provision of a source of simple benefit for the person – being able to de-stress, being able to relax and experiencing some personal healing. However, these experiences can be seductive and lead people into a world which is initially attractive but in time turns dark and dangerous.

When advocates of these practices declare that the practices are not religious they are trying to reassure people that they are not being duped into another religion. Yet, each of these practices has a strong "theological" basis. They carry a vision of the human person and a clear understanding of the nature of the divine. Each of them, in fact, has a spiritual origin and draws practitioners into these religious philosophies. They all offer an alternative understanding of the make-up of the human person and they invite people to discover their view of the divine reality.

By their nature they do not stop with the simple physical exercises – their advocates know the deeper spiritual meaning of what they are doing. They can't help but promote this deeper reality. They want to lead people to the truth as they see it. Thus people are drawn into this new and exotic spiritual realm. This worldview is at odds with Christian faith and belief.

The divine, as they see it, is an impersonal force – and not the personal God revealed in Christianity. The practitioner, fascinated with the discovery of new powers, is drawn to surrender to this divine force. Simple exercises of relaxation can lead to idolatry!

As a priest and bishop I have met with many cases of people who now suffer from terrible spiritual afflictions which are clearly linked to their participation in these practices. In innocence and curiosity they have pursued an interest in these systems and have found themselves trapped in a world of dark and destructive forces. This book provides a much needed warning.

On two particular occasions the Catholic Church has addressed questions associated with the use of techniques taken from Eastern religions. In 1989 the then Cardinal Ratzinger as Prefect of the Congregation for the Doctrine of the Faith published *Some Aspects of Christian Meditation* and in 2002 the Pontifical Council for Culture and the Pontifical Council for Interreligious Dialogue combined to produce a reflection on the New Age, entitled *Jesus Christ, the Bearer of the Water of Life.*

In the first of these documents the methods of meditation used by Eastern religions were compared with the Catholic tradition of meditation. The document warns of dangers associated with embracing Eastern forms of meditation which may threaten the integrity of Christian prayer.

The second document contrasts New Age religiosity with Christian faith. It points to the difference between the Christian's faith in a personal God revealed in Jesus Christ with impersonal energies proposed in various New Age spiritualities. It asks the question: "Is God a being with whom we have a relationship or something to be used or a force to be harnessed?"

Brother Max Sculley in this book addresses these questions by revealing clearly that what underpins these techniques is quite foreign to Christianity and damaging to the faith and possibly the life of the practitioner.

This book is timely. The research into the background to these techniques raises many questions. With the widespread use of these practices and with many Catholics attracted to their use this book provides a very valuable service in warning of the dangers associated with embracing the underlying philosophies to these practices.

The book recounts many examples of people who have found

themselves seriously threatened by powerful and destructive spiritual forces as a result of embracing these techniques.

For the Christian the spiritual life is an engagement with the Holy Spirit. This Spirit offers the pure water of saving grace. The Catholic tradition is rich in experience and teaching in the ways of the spiritual life. We have the example of the great mystics and a library of spiritual writings that offer wisdom, insight and sure guidance for anyone wishing to enter more deeply into the divine life offered through faith in Jesus Christ, who is the "bearer of the water of life".

Julian Porteous
Auxiliary Bishop of Sydney
9 April 2011

Preface

For 25 years one of the constants in my life has been involvement in Christian adult education, mostly with Catholics but also on occasion with Protestants. My focus has been on positive aspects of Christianity – re-evangelising, teaching the word of God, forms of Christian meditation and equipping lay people for ministry in the Church. In more recent times, however, I have become increasingly preoccupied by the rapidly growing number of Christians becoming involved in 'energy practices' such as yoga, tai chi and Reiki. I have also become increasingly aware of members of my own Church, including priests, religious and laity, flocking to the yoga gurus, tai chi masters and Reiki practitioners, and that practices/classes are sometimes available in Catholic institutions.

Leaders in my own Church have remained largely silent about the phenomenon. Even the Vatican publication, *Jesus Christ the Bearer of the Water of Life*,[1] a commentary on New Age, evoked little response from local Church leaders in regard to these three practices which nestle comfortably into New Age. Some Catholics, rightly or wrongly, may interpret such silence as assent.

In the light of this, I decided to write a comprehensive critique of yoga, tai chi and Reiki from a Christian perspective. My hope is that much of what I have written will also be acceptable to my Protestant friends since it is based largely on the word of God and quotes many Protestant writers.

Why these three energy systems? Enormous numbers of people in society are flocking to each of them. There is a remarkable similarity in the belief systems underlying each, all involve techniques which produce altered states of consciousness,[2] and all of them at the advanced stage can result in the achievement of occult powers and even supposed divinisation. What is particularly striking, at the heart of each religious belief system is the worship of an impersonal god so vastly different from the personal God of Christianity whose outstanding characteristic is loving mercy as witnessed by the life, death and resurrection of Jesus and encapsulated so beautifully in the parable of the Prodigal Father.[3] This biblical emphasis on the mercy of God is very much reinforced and amplified in the book, *Divine Mercy in My Soul, Diary of St Maria Faustina Kowalska.*[4]

Altered States of Consciousness (ASC)

A recurring refrain in our treatment of these three energy systems is the creation of abnormal mental states by a variety of techniques. Such mental states are commonly referred to as 'Altered States of Consciousness' which lie at the heart of New Age spirituality. Such states are generally characterised by a significant reduction of logical thought and passivity of will.

The term ASC does not include altered mental states which characterise day-dreaming, sleeping and dreaming which form part of the natural cycle of human life. Nor does it apply to genuine Christian or biblical mystical experiences such as visions, ecstasies or prophetic revelations. Such experiences differ from ASCs in that these altered states are not produced by human techniques but happen spontaneously and unbidden by the direct action of the Holy Spirit. They result in a world view and a morality in accord with biblical and Christian tradition; they generally help to build up the People of God in their faith, and recipients of such revelations glorify, not themselves or demonic spirits, but the one true God.

In the text, we outline the different ways in which ASCs are induced in our three energy systems. But as is well known, there are numerous other ways of inducing an ASC, as for example through zen meditation, hypnosis,[5] shamanic trance-dances, certain types of visualisation, centring prayer and the ingestion of mind-altering drugs such as mescaline and LSD.[6]

Adepts of ASCs commonly experience a sense of oneness with the cosmos and with the divine and may even come to believe that they are divine through the feelings of bliss and the psychic powers they experience. They may experience revelations through visions and often experience a restructuring of their world view.

The dangers which may result from ASC practice are mental illness, demonic influence, spirit possession and occult bondage. The term 'occult' as used in this book, unless otherwise indicated, means 'related to demonic influence'.

Ankerberg and Weldon who treat the topic of ASCs extremely well in their *Encyclopedia of New Age Beliefs*,[7] provide ample evidence to show that such mind-altering techniques may expose one to a range of demonic spirits which lead one into beliefs and practices contrary to biblical teaching.

One case-study to which Ankerberg and Weldon draw our attention may give us pause to consider the dangers associated with profoundly altered states of consciousness. Carl was a leading parapsychologist practising as a professor in a university in Mid-Western USA. An Episcopalian very interested in Christianity, he was convinced that over the centuries it had been corrupted by the churches. He had a strong desire to discover primitive Christianity and sought to do this by transcending the boundaries of time through altered states of consciousness. He claimed to be able to enter into past life experiences through astral travel and communicated these experiences to his amazed students.

As his psychic powers became stronger and his mystical experiences grew more profound, he began to notice changes in his personality. At one period, he began to have misgivings about the path he was following but quickly suppressed these. Eventually, evil forces operating within him caused a serious breakdown and left him 'an incoherent shell of a man'.[8] He underwent a very difficult but successful exorcism and 11 months of hospitalisation. After his recovery, he wrote a letter to his large following of disciples and confessed:

> Solemnly and of my own free will I wish to acknowledge that knowingly and freely I entered into possession by an evil spirit. And although that spirit came under the guise of saving me, perfecting me, helping me to help others, I knew all along it was evil.[9]

Then Carl went on to outline the cause of his demise:

> My central error, which was both intellectual and moral in character, concerned the nature of human consciousness. Like many before me and many others nowadays, I found that with rigid and expert training I could attain a fascinating state of consciousness, a complete absence of any particular object (in my awareness). I found I could attain a permanency on this plane of consciousness.[10]

Such are the dangers of practising ASCs in a disciplined way over an extended period of time.

Many Christians who practise yoga and tai chi seek to distance themselves from the pagan system of beliefs underlying each. What they fail to realise is that the mind-altering techniques which are an integral part of these practices, by themselves alone, present serious spiritual risks.

My sincere hope and prayer is that this book may alert Christians, and indeed all people of good will, to the dangers hidden beneath the surface of these apparently innocent and healing arts. May those who have been already seduced by the sensations of bliss and occult powers gained through them, come, through the Blood and Water which flowed from the All-merciful Heart of Jesus,[11] to that experience of the love of the one true God which surpasses all comprehension.

Part A

YOGA

1

Out of India

Fifty years ago, yoga was relatively unknown in Australia. But with the increased emphasis on good health, the rise of alternative medical treatments, increased stress in our society and the emergence of New Age practices, yoga has risen dramatically in popularity around the Western world. It now ranks as the tenth most common form of exercise in this country. It is rare to find a suburb or country town where yoga classes are not offered. Sessions are held on TV, and videos and DVDs produced by yoga teachers are readily available. Perhaps the greatest promoter of it, as of many things New Age, is the Theosophical Society through its global network of bookshops and libraries. Even tabloid newspapers get into the act, offering free DVDs on yoga.

Recently I was talking to a young married woman who had been advised by her naturopath to take up yoga. As nearly all her friends had taken it up for health reasons or to cope with stress, the temptation to do so was strong. However, as a person whose Christianity defines her life, she came to me seeking guidance. As you read this book you will learn what my advice was.

Yoga, for the most part imported from India, is commonly marketed in Australia as a means of reducing stress and improving one's physical, emotional and spiritual health. At least 45 different types of yoga are practised here and 80 per cent of yoga practitioners are female. The numerous branches of yoga may be broadly classified under two categories, hatha yoga and raja yoga

A third manifestation, Kundalini yoga, is common to all forms of yoga. Kundalini, meaning coiled like a snake, is the arousal of psycho-spiritual energy. It is treated more fully later.

The common attitude towards yoga, especially hatha yoga, is that it is "perfectly OK". Some would add: "It's all about spirituality and not about religion". In response, the thesis of this book is:

1. **Yoga imported from India is inextricably linked to the religious beliefs of Hinduism.**
2. **The key beliefs of Hinduism clash head-on with the beliefs of Christians.**
3. **Altering one's state of consciousness, a practice common to all yogas, is highly dangerous as it can easily open up the mind to demonic influences and may result in occult powers, a number of which are specifically condemned in the Bible.**

Out of India

Most forms of yoga (including hatha and raja) are imports from India. They derive from philosophy based on the Vedas, the oldest scriptures of Hinduism dating back to 1500 BC, referred to as Vedantic philosophy. French Benedictine Dechanet has summed up the Westernised yoga based on this philosophy correctly: "It is a brahmanised yoga, where Hinduism has soaked into the marrow of its bones; it is a yoga enslaved to a system of thought entirely Indian and Vedantist".[1]

Vedantist philosophy is basically a system of religious beliefs which answers the following questions:

- Who made the world?
- How was the world made?
- What is the purpose of life?

• Do humans have a soul/spirit?

• How does one obtain 'supernatural powers'?

• What is the morally good life?

• How can one be delivered from deeds which harm the self and the punishment which goes with such deeds?

• What happens after death?

• How does one obtain happiness in this life and the next?

• How can one make contact with the spirit world?

Hatha Yoga

Hatha or physical yoga is the form of yoga most commonly practised in Australia. It involves:

  • a series of poses performed in silence
  • controlled, slow, rhythmic breathing
  • focusing of the mind on the bodily movements and the breathing
  • repetition of a mantra.

The retarded breathing, allegedly, is a powerful means of absorbing prana (divine energy) from the air, circulating it through the body and storing it. The poses performed slowly, the rhythmic and slow breathing, and the repetition of a mantra are all easy means of entering into an altered state of consciousness.

In such states, the practitioner learns to feel the prana within the body and to direct it to different parts of the body using willpower and visualisation techniques. Through prana stored in the body at different chakras (energy centres), yogis may become capable of transferring healing power by touch to a sick person. The famous 'shaktipat' or 'blessing of a guru', involves the guru touching the initiate on the head and thus transmitting a powerful surge of prana through the head to the whole body.

The peak of achievement is reached when the mind becomes a void for extended periods. At this stage, the yogi enters a state of self-realisation or enlightenment, becoming aware that (s)he is divine

?
*

and completely at one with the cosmos. The sense that one is a god is strongly nourished by a host of psychic powers which accompany this stage. The rousing of the kundalini, though fraught with hazards, is regarded as a powerful means of hastening this enlightenment process.

Raja Yoga

This is similar to hatha yoga in its:

- physical poses
- retarded breathing
- use of a mantra
- the rousing of the kundalini

It differs from hatha yoga in its highly refined techniques of concentration and meditation, the mastering of which results in profoundly altered states of consciousness and numerous psychic powers.

In the West, both hatha and raja yoga study are commonly based on non-dualistic Vedantic philosophy, a Hindu philosophy 'uncompromising in its monistic and pantheistic views; Brahman is All and the only Reality; all else is illusion'.[2]

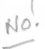

The ultimate purpose of both hatha and raja is the same — the realisation of one's own divinity, a concept utterly at odds with Christianity.

The Seven Major Chakras

Chakras, sometimes called energy centres, are 'depots' of concentrated prana (see **Figure One** next page).

In kundalini yoga, prana is believed to rise from the base chakra and to gradually pass through the spine to all the higher chakras till it reaches the crown chakra.

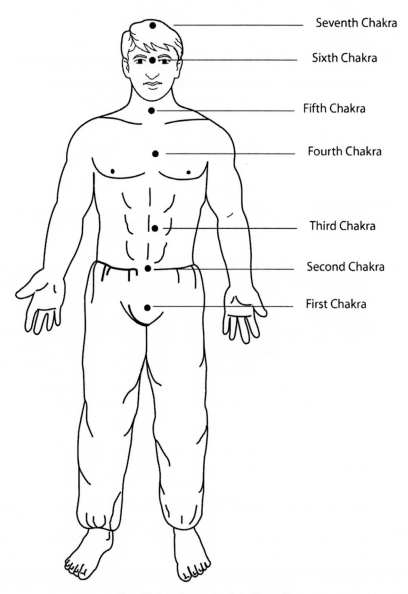

Seventh Chakra

Sixth Chakra

Fifth Chakra

Fourth Chakra

Third Chakra

Second Chakra

First Chakra

Graphic based on a sketch by Kevin Tan

Arousing the Kundalini

'Kundalini', a Hindu goddess popularised by tantric yoga, is represented as a coiled snake sleeping at the base of the spine. This snake is metaphorically pictured as rising up the spine and being finally united at the crown chakra with her consort, the Hindu god Shiva.

This process is regarded by yoga authorities such as Svatmarama and Gopi Krishna as extremely dangerous and may result in illness, insanity or even death, especially if attempted without a guru. Gopi Krishna himself had close brushes with insanity and death.[3]

The process is:

- common to all forms of yoga including Buddhist, Sufi, Bede Griffith's Hybrid Yoga and Dechanet's so-called Christian Yoga;

- particularly popularised in the West by converts to Tantric Yoga in which 'sex… is not used primarily for pleasure, but rather for spiritual enlightenment';[4]

- involves the transfer of large amounts of sexual pranic energy from the base chakra through the hollow canal in the middle of the spine. As the 'divine energy' moves upwards and reaches different chakras, the practitioner receives certain psychic powers appropriate to each chakra;

- these psychic powers, include the ability to read a person's mind, be aware of so-called past lives, the ability to communicate with the spirit world including 'gods', 'angels', the souls of the dead, clairvoyancy, levitation, healing, astral projection and visions;

- when, after much practice, the prana reaches the crown chakra, the adept becomes enlightened or self-realised and is now, supposedly, divine;

- at this point the yogi is now totally karma-free and will no more be reincarnated after death – he or she is supposedly immortal.[5]

In terms of the kundalini process, the following observation is worthy of note: 'A yoga teacher for ten years and a former vice-principal of a large yoga school, and now a Christian, said: **Every posture is designed to stimulate kundalini.**'[6] Note that such stimulation is normally facilitated by an ASC brought about through retarded breathing which is intrinsic to Western yoga.

Just a Health Kick?

In Australia today, hatha yoga is big business and is seen by the health profession, the populace and by many Christian pastors as a sound means of gaining good physical and emotional health. To consider it psychologically or spiritually harmful is generally regarded as erroneous and alarmist.

Yet a few documented examples of people who have been harmed, some critically, by their involvement in so-called 'innocent' hatha yoga, however, challenge the popular misconception that hatha yoga is harmless.

Christina Grof

Christina, now a New Age celebrity, was prior to her experience of a form of hatha yoga, an average housewife with no unusual plans for her life. Since it is widely claimed that 'during pregnancy, yoga exercises are extremely beneficial and will keep you supple and relaxed',[7] Christina decided to take up a variation of yoga when she fell pregnant with her first child. However, in submitting herself to this common form of pre-natal preparation which involves the retarded breathing as practised in hatha yoga, she got far more than she expected as she wrote in *The Yoga Journal* (USA):

> During the birth of my first child, for which I had prepared with the Lamaze method of breathing, this enormous spiritual force was released in me. Of course, I didn't understand it and was given

morphine to stop it as soon as the baby was born. This all led to more and more experiences. I threw myself into yoga, although still not acknowledging it as a spiritual tool. My meeting with Swami Muktananda really blew the lid off everything. He served as a catalyst to awaken what I had been resisting, which was kundalini.[8]

As sometimes happens with kundalini yoga, symptoms of a mental breakdown began to appear. Grof became increasingly convinced she was going mad: 'I was convinced I was headed for a life of psychopathology. I was afraid I was going crazy.'[9]

Nevertheless, she claims counselling through yogic philosophy helped put matters in their 'proper' perspective. Her marriage broke up and the late popular mythologist and Jungian psychologist Joseph Campbell helped her recognise 'the schizophrenic is drowning in the same waters in which the mystic is swimming with delight'.[10] He also suggested she take LSD and referred her to consciousness researcher Stan Grof for more counselling.

She married Grof and the couple have since become leaders in New Age, coordinating some 50 Emergency Centres around the world. In doing so, they have become expert at re-interpreting pathologies induced by occult practice as 'transforming spiritualities', thus clouding the whole discernment process:

> For example, in the case of kundalini yoga, symptoms of mental illness and demonisation are gratuitously defined as emerging manifestations of 'higher' or divine consciousness. Thus we are not to question or fear the kundalini process but to surrender to it and trust it implicitly, for it is part of an ageless wisdom of evolutionary transformation which is far wiser than ourselves.[11]

It is worthy of note that in their book *Spiritual Emergency*, one chapter is headed 'When Insanity Is a Blessing.'[12]

Thus, in the long run, Christina Grof's flirtation with a hatha yoga technique altered her whole life and resulted in her becoming a New Age guru, with influence over hundreds of thousands of people.

Carole

Carole tells her story in *The Coming Darkness: Confronting Occult Deception*.[13] Carole turned to yoga for health reasons. She was very sick and doctors were unable to find the cause. When she went to a physician–nutritionist recommended by a friend, she found some literature in his office about the Himalayan Institute, of which the doctor was a member. The Institute was founded by Indian Swami Rama, one of the most scientifically studied of the gurus. Carole decided to attend the institute in the U.S.A. where she began lessons in hatha yoga. Eventually she was initiated and received her mantra from Swami Rama.[14] As Rama laid his hands upon her head to give the guru's traditional blessing or 'shaktipat', the characteristic transfer of occult energy began and Carole experienced utter bliss:

> Currents of electrical energy began to permeate my head and went down into my body ... It was as if a spell had come over me, the bliss that I felt was as if I had been touched by God. The power that had come from his hand, and simply being in his presence, drew me to him irresistibly.[15]

The following night she was visited by a spirit-entity which 'claimed to be the spirit of Swami Rama himself. Carole felt that she was communing directly with God.'[16] As Carole describes it:

> Electrical currents were pulsating around my body, and then moved into my hand. The currents were shaking my hand and strong, almost entrancing thoughts were impressed into my mind, 'Meditate, meditate, I want to speak with you.' It was a miracle. I was communicating with the spirit world I had found. Sitting in the darkness of my living room I began to repeat my mantra. A presence seemed to fill the room. I began to see visions of being one with the universe and the magnetic thoughts were now leaving and I was hearing a voice which identified itself as Swami Rama, saying he was communicating with me through astral travel.

> Within one week after meditating many hours each day and still
> in constant communication with this spirit, forces began to come
> upon me and gave me power to do yoga postures. I was floating
> through them, the forces giving me added breath even ... postures
> that before would be very painful to do.[17]

However, after two weeks of daily yoga meditation, the honeymoon
was over. Carole became engulfed in an occult nightmare of utter
terror. Voices that once claimed they were angelic, now turned
threatening, even demonic. She was brutally assaulted both physically
and spiritually by spirits.[18] She was subjected to constant attacks from
her spirits whom she felt were seeking to kill her. In desperation she
consulted a string of doctors, psychologists and spiritualists to no
avail. In fact, one spiritualist 'admitted that Carole's situation was not
uncommon among followers of Eastern gurus,' and he even reported
to her that sometimes death follows such attacks.[19]

When Carole was on the point of death, a series of events resulted
in her becoming a Christian. Jesus freed her totally from her torments,
and much to the amazement of her psychiatrist, she is now in perfect
health both mentally and physically. All of Carole's problems had
begun with a simple course in hatha yoga.

A Vicar's Wife

Brenda Skyrme, an experienced Christian counsellor in England,
narrates in her book, *Martial Arts and Yoga*, how a vicar's wife presented
herself to Brenda for help. For some time she had been unable to
make any sense out of her daily Bible readings:

> All her life she had been a keen Bible student and suddenly and
> only recently the words meant nothing to her any more. She was
> suffering from confusion in every area of her Christian life. She
> had even lost her customary ability to pray spontaneously at the
> Mothers' Union meetings. Every part of her church work had
> become an effort.[20]

Earlier, her husband had agreed to rent out the church hall for a yoga class, and several of the congregation, including the vicar's wife, had decided to attend. It was after the class that her difficulties commenced. At first she couldn't believe something as apparently harmless as yoga could have affected her, but after an explanation of the background to yoga and some ministry,[21] she was freed from the oppression that had affected her and 'she returned home with great joy'.[22]

Innocent Hatha Yoga Kundalini?

We have given three examples of people who had limited exposure to Hatha Yoga. This is not to say that all who take part in this form of yoga experience the same negative effects as these persons. I spoke to a number of people who had taken part in this form of yoga and who claimed to have experienced no ill effects, psychological or spiritual. It could be that some of these had a subtle tarnishing of their spirit of which they were unaware. **However, the point we are making here is that anyone, even those who lay no claim to the religious elements of such yoga, are putting themselves at risk by taking part in activities such as retarded breathing and the repetition of a mantra, both of which practices are specifically designed to induce an ASC which exposes one to demonic influence.**

What is even more dangerous in Australia at present, hatha yoga is being increasingly used to produce the kundalini awakening. This, as with Christina and Carol, may be triggered simply by the 'guru's blessing' at initiation and then further developed by certain techniques practised in hatha yoga, in which, as we have pointed out, 'Every posture is designed to stimulate kundalini'. Apart from being psychologically risky, as Hindu authorities tell us, kundalini arousal commonly leads to such psychic powers as contact with the 'spirits of the dead' leading to clairvoyance and awareness of 'past lives', practices in conflict with biblical teaching.

In this connection, it is interesting to note that Christina Grof in concert with her husband, set up a network of some 50 centres around the world to assist people who were going through 'personal transformation crises' through altered states of consciousness. They reported that 'one fourth of our callers are experiencing manifestations of Kundalini awakening.'[23] That was back in 1989. Since then, kundalini arousal yoked with hatha yoga has spread much more widely in the West.

Another point worthy of note in all this is the spiritualist-counsellor's observation to Carole that 'her situation was not uncommon among followers of Eastern gurus'. So in referring to Christina and Carole, we are not referring to isolated cases.

A Glimpse at Raja Yoga

Mary, who dabbled in raja yoga wrote this account for publication:

> I had always been interested in psychic phenomena and the power of healing through deep tissue massage with oils, and the laying of hands. So when an acquaintance said that I had the power of healing and asked me if I would like to go with her to a meeting at the Spiritualist Church, I said 'Why not?'
>
> The speaker was a doctor from San Francisco who gave an interesting talk on the benefits of using crystals for healing. He stressed the fact that the crystal was just a tool, the power and the energy come from the healer through it.
>
> Then after reading Deepak Chopra and viewing some of his videos on raja yoga, I became mesmerised by the wonder of it all.
>
> I just had to find that perfect healing crystal and learn to meditate, for meditation seemed to be the key to unlock the mystery of this New Age phenomenon.
>
> After joining a yoga class I learned how to relax the mind. And I enjoyed visualising myself at my beautiful private place which was a lush grassy area with a waterfall tumbling down into a beautiful violet-coloured pool.

With practice I mastered the art of falling asleep in one minute at night. Although I must say this. After buying my special crystal, after some sleepless nights I discovered I could not sleep without it in my room.

After receiving my mantra from the local Transcendental Meditation Centre, I became quite adept at meditation, but after a while I found myself being abruptly woken at three o'clock every morning and the same female person's face was there in front of me. Then I noticed that while in deep meditation periods the white light that we always sought seemed to be getting darker and noisier. And at work my feelings for one particular workmate, the one whose face appeared to me at night, were getting, can I say, unhealthy. I thought: what is happening here? I am a married woman with a loving husband and family. My whole sexual identity seemed to have turned upside down. I found myself admiring beautiful women instead of handsome men. By this time I was right into affirmations of telling myself how great I was. And then you tell yourself that you are God.

That was, I suppose, when I woke up. I knew it was time to reclaim my former life. I packed all my New Age and yoga stuff in a bag and threw them into the harbour where they could not harm anyone again.

My thoughts on this experience are that while our minds are empty, we surrender our bodies to demonic spirits like Lesbos, and because it feels at the time so wonderful and euphoric, we tell ourselves it must be good, it can't be evil. I did go through a long period of depression after this, but with the help of our Blessed Lord and Our Lady, I came through.

Yoga's inroads into the mainstream

Open many popular magazines, look at the noticeboard at many gyms or even the noticeboard at many workplaces that offer health advice to staff and yoga is prominently promoted. The practice has become so fashionable that even many top level professional football clubs are getting involved and talking enthusiastically about the positive benefits. Years ago it became the fashion in top level football circles to gain that extra edge in positive thinking by having hypnotism sessions before the game. All sorts of claims were made for its success. That fashion soon faded. The interesting feature common to both hypnosis and yoga meditation is that they both involve altered states of consciousness.

Yoga Invades the Church

It is not merely the secular worlds of sport and health that have been captivated by yoga. Some few years ago I chanced upon a news sheet at the back of a Catholic church in outer south-western Sydney, entitled *Family Watch* (Issue 15). Its publisher was Catholic Church Insurances Ltd. According to the accompanying article, *Balancing Body and Mind: Finding energy to 'seize the day' as they say can sometimes be an uphill battle. That's why more and more Australians are turning to time-honoured practices such as yoga, meditation, tai chi and qigong to help them unwind and de-stress.*[24]

The fine print under the photo made it clear that the class was practising not yoga but a Chinese variant called 'qigong' (pronounced chi kung) which the instructor described as a cross between tai chi and yoga. The article enthusiastically listed numerous health benefits which purportedly result from chi kung, concluding that it also 'promotes happiness and peace of mind'.[25] And should the Catholic in the pew still have had any lingering doubts, we were reassured by the testimony of the converted: *Enlightened staff members at Catholic Church Insurances have discovered this for themselves after attending a short course in chi kung relaxation techniques run earlier in the year.*[26]

Websites on tai chi, chi kung and yoga were provided. It appeared that Catholic Church Insurances were keen to see the number of the 'enlightened' increase.

But it would be a mistake to think that the spreading of the good news of yoga is limited only to the business arm of the Church. Many Christian churches throughout the country let their halls/ retreat centres for yoga classes, in which parishioners/retreatants participate. At times, teachers in Catholic high schools who practise yoga themselves may take a yoga video or DVD into a class to show the students, or run some yoga classes during the last two weeks of school when normal classes have slackened off.

Most people in society and in our Christian churches would say, 'So what?' They would echo the cry of the promoters of yoga — 'yoga can be practised by people of any religion. It is based on an ancient wisdom at the heart of all religions and acceptable to them all. It is based on a philosophy and is not a religion'.

2

The Philosophy of Yoga

The great masters of yoga consistently proclaim that yoga is independent of all religions and will fit any creed. Yoga practices can be followed, they say, with equal benefit by the Hindu, the Muslim, the Buddhist, the Taoist, the free-thinker and the Catholic. Yoga, they insist, is founded on an ancient wisdom upon which all religions are based. However, the guru says to the disciple as (s)he takes the first halting steps along the yogic path: *Don't just accept the word of our Hindu scriptures and writings based on them. Go and verify their truth through your own experience.*

It is the direct experience of the supernatural world which yoga provides that makes it so attractive to people in the West, many of whom have been starved of religious experience.

However, there is one major problem with making such experience the touchstone of truth. The answers provided by yoga experience and which are in accord with Hindu philosophy, for the most part, flatly contradict the answers revealed by Jesus Christ and entrusted to His Church.

Basic Beliefs of Yoga Philosophy

Brahman

The supreme being of Hinduism and hence of yoga is Brahman. Brahman is totally impersonal, infinite energy. It is the creator of all the other Hindu gods who are personal and hence illusory. Brahman is the creator of all things in the universe. But it is not only the creator, it is also its own creation. This means that all creation is but an extension of Brahman. A good illustration of this is the spider that creates its web out of its own saliva, making the web an extension of the spider. Such a belief system is referred to as 'pantheism' and may be summed up in the popular term, 'God is all, all is god'.[1]

Prana

The name commonly given to Brahman as the spiritual essence of all created things is 'prana'. So really prana is cosmic Brahman. In introductory courses in yoga, prana is commonly referred to as 'energy' or 'vital energy', both of which fail to convey the divine nature of prana.

Nature is Divine

Since prana is the divine essence at the heart of all created things, everything in the universe is divine – the sun, moon, stars, the sea, the river, the plants. However, in the mind of the Hindu, some things are seen as being more divine than others. The sun, because it is the richest source of prana in our system is accorded official worship. Amongst animals, the cow and the snake are accorded special worship, as are the rhizome and the lotus among plants.

Make Me Impersonal Like Brahman

In non-dualistic Vedantic yoga belief, the outer nature of all things is illusion. It is only the inner spiritual essence which is divine and that is all that matters. In humans, the outer part is the body and the ego, which includes the emotions, intellect and will. The inner divine essence is the soul, which is the impersonal Brahman. This is sometimes referred to as the Spirit, the Higher Self, or in Hindu terms, Atman. The whole purpose of yoga is to kindle the divine spark within, so that it eventually becomes a blazing fire. For this to occur, the outer part of humans, the body and ego, which are illusory anyway, must be consumed as a holocaust in this divine fire. Moti Lal Pandit, noted Indian scholar of Eastern religions and himself a yogi, informs us that 'the aim of yoga is to realise liberation from the human condition. To achieve this liberation, various psychological, physical, mental and mystical methods have been devised. All these methods are anti-social (sometimes even anti-human) in that yoga prescribes a way of life which says: this mortal life is not worth living.'[2] And finally, one of the leading gurus, Sri Aurobindo, observes: 'We can do very well without the mind ... (and) in truth, we are the better for it.'[3]

The Mirage of Marriage

Swami Yogananda expresses succinctly how the yogi views the world: 'One's values are profoundly changed when he is finally convinced that creation is only a vast motion picture and that not in it, but beyond it, lies his own reality.'[4]

In accordance with this belief the Swami describes marriage as 'a drama'[5] – virtual reality, not the real thing which can only be discovered fully beyond this present life. What is this saying in terms of marriage? Marriage is necessary to satisfy human love and for procreation, but it fades in importance in comparison with the much higher priority of pursuing the things of the spirit both in this life and in the next. For those seriously following the way of yoga, sexual restraint is 'a must' in seeking to arouse the kundalini. It is conserved sexual energy converted into pranic energy which is so powerful in kundalini yoga. Vivekananda, one of the first of the Indian gurus to bring yoga to the West, leaves us in no doubt:

> It is only the chaste man or woman who can make the ojas (high level prana) rise and store it in the brain; that is why chastity has always been considered the highest virtue ... There must be perfect chastity in thought, word and deed; without it the practice of raja yoga is dangerous and may lead to insanity.[6]

The ideal, of course, is to live a celibate life as an Indian monk, a swami, like Vivekananda and Yogananda. If one cannot be a swami, the next best thing is to severely limit one's sexual activity in marriage to brief encounters in order to beget children and then move quickly back into the celibate yoga mode. In India, it has been quite common for more senior fathers, after rearing their children, to retire into solitude to pursue yoga. But such may happen even with younger parents.

This was the case with the parents of Rabi Maharaj, a yogi prodigy who became a guru in his teenage years, and who eventually defected from yoga and Hinduism to become a committed Christian. Both of Rabi's parents became 'lost' in yoga while Rabi was a child. Such examples abound in yogic literature. For example, Yogananda relates that his parents fell under the sway of the great master, Lahiri Mahasaya, becoming his disciples early in their married life. Yogananda gives us a brief glimpse into their sex life, and 'brief' is the operative word here:

Mother made a remarkable admission to my eldest sister: 'Your father and myself live together as man and wife only once a year, for the purpose of having children.'[7] Their brief encounters seem to have been fruitful, for they managed to have eight children!

In his definitive work on yoga, Mircea Eliade sums up the Hindu yogi's attitude to life: *This world is rejected, this life depreciated because it is known that something else exists, beyond becoming, beyond temporality, beyond suffering. In religious terms, it could be said that India rejects the profane cosmos and profane life, because it thirsts for a sacred world and a sacred mode of living.*[8]

Karma and Reincarnation

In accord with Hindu teaching, yogis firmly believe in the doctrines of karma and reincarnation, beliefs that go hand in hand. Karma means literally 'actions'. During a given lifetime, a person performs a mix of deeds, some of which are conducive to one's evolution

towards enlightenment and some of which retard it. If, at the point
of death the karmic balance is positive, one proceeds to complete
liberation from the cycle of rebirthing, and the soul enters eternal
bliss. This, in Hindu teaching, appears to be relatively rare. If the
account balance is negative at the time of death, one is supposedly
condemned by the law of nature's justice, cause and effect, to rebirth
as a human being, as an animal or as an even lower form of life.
The state into which one is born is determined precisely by one's
karmic bank balance. The common opinion is that the great majority
of people end up in hundreds or thousands of rebirths, and that for
some, the reincarnation cycle never ends.

Within the lifespan of an individual, it is also believed that a
negative deed often has negative consequences in the here and now.
Harm may come from another person or from a natural catastrophe.
Similarly, positive deeds may result in positive consequences in this
life.

The concept of karma is based on the law of strict justice. There
is no such thing as forgiveness by Brahman. In Hindu thinking,
the quickest and most effective way of improving one's karmic
bank balance is through yoga, especially raja yoga. Even within the
space of one lifetime, a yogi, so it is alleged, by following a series of
techniques, may reach enlightenment and gain immortal bliss after
death – salvation by the Self.

Because the system is one of strict justice based on an impersonal
god, there is no place for forgiveness on the part of that god and no
dispensation of mercy. This is in complete contrast to Christianity in
which Jesus Christ through his suffering, death and resurrection atones
for our sins, both original and personal. In God's plan as revealed
in Christ, there is only one way of being justified and sanctified —
through repenting of sin and the redeeming power of Jesus. Peter
made this plain when he addressed the Jews after Pentecost: *Only in
Jesus Christ is there salvation, for of all the names in the world given to humans,*

this is the only one by which we can be saved.[9]

Unlike the impersonal god Brahman/Prana, the Christian Trinity is essentially personal – the three Persons, the Father, Son and Holy Spirit in the deepest communion with each other. The Father, in His great love and mercy, sent His Son to redeem the human race from its rebellion, with the most outstanding attribute of God revealed to us in the face of Jesus being His loving mercy. The words of the psalmist: *The Lord is gracious and full of compassion, slow to anger and abounding in mercy and loving kindness,*[10] take flesh in the person of Jesus as He proclaims the parable of the 'Prodigal Father' (Lk 15:11-31) and as He reaches out to sinners, epitomised in the forgiveness of the good thief with his dying breath: 'In truth I tell you, today you will be with me in paradise.'[11]

Minus the Religious Yolk

In promoting yoga, it is not unusual for yoga teachers in the West, at least initially, to bypass the religious system of belief at the heart of the practice, which many adherents remain in ignorance about. What is stressed instead are the 20 basic hatha yoga poses and the promise of health, happiness and peace of mind drawn from an ancient science practised in the East for thousands of years. With the confidence and enthusiasm of evangelists, teachers promise that the practice of the poses will give increased stability, clarity of mind, contentment and capacity for concentration that will enhance all aspects of life.

Doing the Poses

In classes and popular DVDs, students are taught the art of retarded breathing (pranayama) which may be accompanied by the repetition of a sanskrit mantra, the meaning of which is often not disclosed to the student. The pranayama and the mantra accompany the performance of the sequence of poses (asanas) done slowly and gracefully in complete silence. The overall effect of this over a period of 30 minutes is to induce an altered state of consciousness characterised by passivity of intellect and will.

The sequence often concludes with the Corpse Pose, which consists in lying full length on the flat of one's back, with legs relaxed and feet falling outwards. The student relaxes each part of the body in succession, starting with the face and ending up with the feet. Once the body is totally 'softened', recruits are urged to relax and 'surrender'. At this early stage, the teacher may not indicate specifically to whom or to what. A study of yoga makes the answer obvious – to the cosmic prana. And though the teacher may refer to it as 'vital energy', prana is just another name for the supreme god of Hinduism – Brahman, which is a pantheistic, impersonal god and quite different to the God whom Christians worship. Hence recruits are being subtly induced to break the First Commandment: 'I am the Lord your God ...You shall have no other Gods to rival Me.'[12]

A similar kind of deception may occur in the use of the Hindu greeting 'Namahste'. The teacher may address the students at the beginning and end of a session with hands joined in the prayer position and a bow to the class saying, 'Namahste'. For recruits, the meaning for this term is sometimes given as 'I salute you' in place of the meaning given to it in yoga circles: 'I bow to the divine essence that is your true nature'. At a later point along the yoga journey, after the regular practice of yoga has begun to alter their belief system, students may be informed that the goal of hatha yoga is to become divine.

As the current leading guru in the West, Deepak Chopra, informs us: 'It does not require you to believe in a set of principles in order to reap yoga's benefits. On the contrary, **the regular practice of yoga naturally generates a healthy belief system** based upon your direct experience of the world through a more flexible nervous system. **Perform yoga poses on a regular basis, and your mind and emotions will change.**'[13] [emphasis added]

If we believe Chopra, so will your belief system change. Soon you will find yourself believing that all is divine – nature, the sun, your guru and you. This is the 'healthy belief system' of a yogi.

Ankerberg and Weldon sum up the situation well: 'Some yoga teachers who run classes for health reasons act deceptively by making no mention of divinity. They know that their exercises will lead them in this direction whether they are conscious of it or not. Thus they avoid establishing it as a religion and any controversy.'[14]

Blowing the Whistle on Hindu Yoga

While the Christian worships the Trinity, the Hindu yogi believes that humans are but a manifestation of Brahman, that their spirit is Brahman. And so from the earliest stages, the practitioner is taught to repeat the affirmation, 'I am that, I am Brahman'.[15] After attaining enlightenment, the adept will then begin to worship him/herself as god and encourage others to do the same. One of the famous Hindu gurus of the 20th century, Muktananda, described what it was like to become a god:

> I was to reach the summit of man's fortune, which is divine realisation. Once the vehicle of a spiritual traveller's sadhana [journey] has reached this point, it stops there forever. There you may see nothing and hear nothing, but at the same time all is seen and heard, for inside you is the spontaneous conviction that you have attained everything. When an aspirant has reached there, he sits in bliss, sleeps in bliss, walks in bliss, comes and goes in bliss. He lives in an ashram in bliss; his behaviour and actions are blissful. He experiences directly, 'Now I have crossed the ocean of worldly existence'. By virtue of this realisation, he is never agitated. No matter what he is doing, his heart is as calm as the ocean.[16]

From this point, Muktananda began to worship himself and encouraged his disciples to offer him divine homage.

Yoga literature abounds with examples of gurus receiving divine worship. Often, what leads people to become devotees is the direct experience of the guru's psychic powers. Barbara Szandorowska, who came from Canada to visit the famous guru Sai Baba in his Indian ashram told of the initial impact which Baba made upon her:

> I put aside my scepticism and opened myself to whatever would happen. As Sai Baba slowly walked in our direction, for the first time, I was aware of an energy flowing from his body towards me. I experienced an exquisite sensation, as though a gentle current of liquid love was pouring into me, caressing me from head to toe. The current came in tender, loving waves that grew stronger as he approached. They rippled through my body, until they permeated my whole being and enveloped me completely. I was filled with peace, such as I hadn't felt in a long time. Even when he left, the feeling of peace remained. I was awe-struck.
>
> If Sai Baba could touch me so deeply in my place of need, the miracles attributed to him could be equally real. Who was this man and how did he get such power?[17]

Soon after this, Barbara went on to worship Sai Baba as god.

Moving the Prana

Yoga devotees claim to be proficient at experiencing prana and feeling the movement of prana within the body. Using techniques of visualisation and willpower, they claim to be able both to move it to any part of the body and to store it at certain energy centres or chakras. They also claim to be able to transfer it to others by touch for the purpose of healing or to convey 'spiritual blessings'.

Some Christians involved in yoga maintain that prana is really the Holy Spirit of Christianity under a different name. They talk of 'feeling the Holy Spirit'; 'directing the Holy Spirit' to parts of the body especially for self-healing, and of 'imparting the Holy Spirit' by touch. Focusing extensively and introspectively on feeling the movement of energy within one's body, however, does not fit easily into the Catholic tradition of meditation and contemplation which focuses on the word of God and the persons of the Trinity, especially Jesus Christ. The movement in such prayer is spiritually outward, away from the body and the self towards God.

Traditional teaching on prayer warns us not to attach undue importance to consolations, and to pay even less heed to FIF – 'funny internal feelings', which may simply be the consequence of an emotional high. In the Christian tradition of prayer, people are encouraged to seek, not the consolations of God but the God of consolation. It is timely to recall the spiritual life of Mother Teresa of Calcutta who experienced utter darkness in her spirit from the time she founded her Sisters in 1950 to the time she died in 1997. Only she can adequately describe this interior, redemptive desolation:

> Now Father – since '49 or '50 this terrible sense of loss – this untold darkness – this loneliness – this continual longing for God – which gives me that pain deep down in my heart. Darkness is such that I really do not see – neither with my mind nor with my reason. The place of God in my soul is blank. There is no God in me – When the pain of longing is so great – I just long and long for God – and then it is that I feel he does not want me. – Sometimes – I just hear my own heart cry out – 'My God' and nothing else comes – The torture and pain I can't explain.[18]

Yet through such enduring darkness, Mother Teresa manifested in her life an extraordinary compassion and love, especially for the poorest of the poor.

If, as some suggest, we equate prana with the Holy Spirit, then we would have yogis 'controlling' the Holy Spirit by directing the Spirit to different parts of the body by sheer will-power and techniques. This would be particularly true of the arousal of the kundalini, where by certain poses and bodily constrictions, prana is forced directly up the spine. This is in direct conflict with Christian prayer, the whole purpose of which is to let oneself be controlled by the Holy Spirit, as Mother Teresa exemplified so well.

Suspect Psychic Siddhis

The classic yoga authorities – Svatmarama (hatha yoga) and Patanjali (raja yoga) — take it for granted in their writings that the adept on the pathway to enlightenment will experience a range of psychic powers or siddhis. A modern guru might describe these powers as 'superconscious abilities', a Christian observer might describe them as 'supernatural powers', and yoga commentators frequently refer to them as 'occult powers', where 'occult' here is taken to mean 'hidden, mysterious, mystical'. Many yoga authorities strongly warn practitioners not to focus on these powers but rather to focus on becoming enlightened. Some of the psychic powers are:

- clairvoyance
- astral travelling
- healing oneself and others
- mind-reading
- an awareness of one's own or others' 'past lives'
- communication with the spirit world — the dead, spirits, gods
- automatic writing

Yoga authorities link such notions with the awakening of the kundalini. Swami Vivekananda, a noted authority on Patanjali's writings, asserts: *When the yogi becomes perfect, there will be nothing in nature not under his control. If he orders the gods or the souls of the departed to come, they will come at his bidding. All the forces of nature will obey him as slaves.*[19]

Such views of yoga authorities are confirmed by the experience of the ex-guru Rabi Maharaj. He noted that certain drugs, by altering the state of consciousness, can produce similar effects to yoga. He described his experience with drug addicts in London after travelling there from India:

I began to encounter increasing numbers of drug addicts and made a startling discovery: some of them were having the same experiences on drugs that I had had in yoga and meditation. I listened in amazement as they described the 'beautiful and peaceful world' they often entered through LSD, a world whose psychedelic sights and sounds were all too familiar to me ... I didn't need drugs to have visions of other worlds and weird beings, and to see the psychedelic colours and to sense a oneness with the universe and the feeling that I was God. I would tell them, 'I got it all by transcendental meditation [as a part of yoga]. **But it was a lie, a trick of evil spirits who took over my mind when I relaxed control of it. You're being deceived. The only way to find the peace and fulfilment you seek is through Christ.**[20] [emphasis added]

Maharaj's experience is worthy of emphasis. Simply by altering their state of consciousness on a regular basis, these drug addicts experienced a change of worldview so that they now perceived themselves as divine and one with the universe. **Some Christians who take up yoga maintain it can do them no harm because they reject the Hindu philosophy underlying it. But in retarding their breathing, they enter into an altered state of consciousness which opens them up to demonic influence which commonly leads to belief in an impersonal god in which all is one (monism), in which god is all (pantheism) and in which the self becomes god. Ironically, this is an expression of Hinduism.**

3

From the Holy Spirit?

A number of the psychic powers or siddhis are roundly condemned by the word of God as interpreted by the Catholic Tradition. In Deuteronomy 18:10-12 we read [the powers in bold print are commonly experienced by yogis]: *Let there be not found among you one who immolates his son or daughter in the fire, not a **fortune-teller, soothsayer, charmer, diviner** or caster of spells, nor one who **consults ghosts or spirits or seeks oracles from the dead**. Anyone who does such things is an abomination to the Lord.*

The *Catechism of the Catholic Church* explains:

> All forms of divination [foretelling the future] are to be rejected:
> recourse to Satan or demons, conjuring up the dead or other
> practices falsely supposed to 'unveil the future'... The phenomena
> of clairvoyance and recourse to mediums all conceal a desire for
> power over time, history, and in the last analysis, other human
> beings, as well as a wish to conciliate hidden powers. They contradict
> the honour, respect and loving fear we owe to god alone.[1]

We have seen that such psychic powers are commonly produced through yoga. One factor involved is the altered state of consciousness of the practitioner. This is compounded by the invocation of false gods such as Brahman, Kundalini and the Self. Mantras given to yoga initiates are frequently the names of such false deities. St Paul, in warning the Corinthians about the dangers of worshipping idols, set them straight about the true nature of such worship:

41

Does this mean that the food sacrificed to idols has a real value, or that the idol itself is real. Not at all. It simply means that the sacrifices they offer, they sacrifice to demons who are not God. I have no desire to see you in communion with demons. You cannot drink the cup of the Lord and the cup of demons.[2]

Paul's words take flesh today in the testimony of Father Rufus Pereira, a highly educated seminary professor, a deliverance minister and exorcist, highly regarded by the Indian Catholic Bishops. Over a period of two years, Fr Pereira prayed to free four hundred individuals from demonic influence. 'He estimated that about a third of them were delivered from demons identifying themselves as Hindu gods.'[3] In one interview, Fr Pereira said:

I love my country very much and have a great respect for Indian religion, but perhaps there is no religion that has within itself such a wide spectrum, ranging all the way from the highest form of religious endeavour to the lowest degradation of humanity – all in the name of religion. I have been led to believe that many of the gods and goddesses in Hindu mythology are nothing other than demons.[4]

He illustrated his point by referring to a young Catholic woman who 'manifested' during a spiritual conference. She was 'stretched out on a table, assuming the dancing posture you see in some Hindu statues. If you tried to straighten her out, she would immediately contort her body back into its artificial posture.'[5] Fr Pereira interpreted the meaning of this manifestation:

You will remember what she looked like, this girl taking on the poses of the Hindu dancing god. (This dancing god is one aspect of the god Shiva.) What is really remarkable is that this girl knows nothing about Indian dancing, because she was brought up in a Western culture home. Yet here she was, assuming the absolutely correct dancing poses in her fingers, her wrists, her hands and feet – the exact poses of this very god. It was something fantastic to watch, as her eyes and her mouth were all changed into the features of this Hindu god. I later found that it got into her because of a spell cast by a Hindu doctor (who perhaps had lustful motives when he was treating her). Probably he called up his favourite god, the dancing god, to possess her so he could get power over her.[6]

Hindu yoga provides a 'double whammy' effect – an exposure to hidden powers or demons through altered states of consciousness and communion with demons through idolatry.

Karma Cleansing Without Christ

The loving mercy of the Christian God seems to be singularly lacking in the visions which our child-yogi Rabi Maharaj experienced: *In my yogic trances most often I would be alone with Shiva the Destroyer sitting fearfully at his feet, the huge cobra [Kali = Kundalini] coiled about his neck staring at me, hissing and darting out its tongue threateningly. Sometimes I wondered why none of the gods I ever encountered seemed kind and gentle and loving.*[7]

Could it be that the Hindu gods that Rabi experienced were but manifestations of demonic spirits as he himself was later to claim after becoming a Christian.

It has been said with some truth that people tend to become like the gods they worship. So if people worship an impersonal god like Brahman, incapable of expressing love and mercy, they tend to behave likewise. So it was not surprising to learn that when Rabi, his relatives and friends converted from Hinduism to Christianity, a marked softening took place among them all, manifested in a willingness to forgive each other and to say 'sorry'.

Karmic Conscience

The law of Karma can at times render the bystander fatalistic and morally inert. Rabi Maharaj highlighted this when he recalled an incident he experienced as a boy while he was being formed as a yogi in a Hindu temple. He was under the tutelage of a swami who was by profession celibate. After some time, it finally dawned on him that the young swami was having an affair with an attractive young woman who frequented the temple. Rabi narrates his experience of people's reaction to the scandal:

> Having admired this brilliant young Brahmin, I was now badly disillusioned and troubled. One day I overheard several regular worshippers discussing the affair in Hindi as they squatted in a tight group on the packed earth of the courtyard. 'This is a private matter – we better not meddle in it', said one handsome man in his forties. An older, white haired man with a long beard, whom I had seen often at the temple, nodded gravely.
>
> 'Of course its karma. They have something of their past life to work out together.' There were sounds of assent and heads nodded in agreement. It made me feel better.[8]

As a result of this collective karma compliance, no action was taken by anyone to alert the temple authorities and so put a stop to the swami's hypocritical immorality. One could object that celibate leaders in the Catholic Church have been guilty of similar offences, and that Church authorities have on occasion turned a blind eye, allowing immorality to persist. Sadly, this is all too true. But the cover-up has generally been due to moral weakness on the part of the authorities. It does not stem in any way from their Catholic religious beliefs.

Karma Courts Continuing Incarnations

While I was researching this book, I spoke with a woman I had known years before as a devout Christian. At the time I contacted her, she was conducting physical fitness classes. I raised the matter of tai chi and she told me that she conducted tai chi sessions for the patients of a Chinese doctor. She hastened to add, *I teach the movements only as exercises and don't go into the philosophy behind it.*' Then she added with some conviction: *I certainly believe in reincarnation though!*

My friend would be one of many Australians who now believe in reincarnation. Christians have compelling reasons for denying reincarnation. Biblical teaching makes it quite clear that we have only one life here on earth: **'Since human beings die only once, after which comes judgement...'** (Heb 9:27) And the parable (Lk 16:19-31), which describes Lazarus going straight to 'Abraham's bosom' and the rich man going to hell straight after death, clearly implies that we have only one life on this earth and this is followed immediately by a personal judgement.

It is on the basis of such texts, as well as the Church's Tradition, that the *Catholic Catechism* teaches: *Each man receives his eternal retribution in his immortal soul at the very moment of his death, in a particular judgement that refers his life to Christ: either entrance into the blessedness of heaven – through a purification or immediately – or immediate and everlasting damnation.*[9]

Jesus Christ – Avatar or Lord?

In Hindu belief, an avatar is the incarnation of a personal god in human form. The Hindu pantheon of avatars includes Rama, Patanjali, Krishna, Buddha and Christ. The latest self-proclaimed avatar is Sai Baba, supposedly the incarnation [in Christian terms] of God the Father. In presenting Jesus Christ on a par with all other avatars, Hinduism clashes with Christianity which reveals that only one God has ever become flesh, the Son of God who incarnated only once in the person of Jesus Christ and who is thereby the unique Lord of all creation:

> And for this God raised [Jesus] on high and gave him the name which above all other names; so that all beings in the heavens, on the earth and in the underworld should bend the knee at the name of Jesus and that every tongue should acknowledge Jesus Christ as Lord, to the glory of God the Father.[10]

Mantras

Ex-guru, Rabi Maharaj, defines the occult nature of the yoga mantra:

> A sound symbol of one or more syllables often used to induce a mystical state. It must be passed on by the living voice of the guru and cannot be learned in another way. One need not understand the meaning of the mantra; the virtue is in the repetition of the sound. **It is said to embody a spirit or deity, and the repetition of the mantra calls this being to the one repeating it**. Thus the mantra both invites a particular being to enter the one using it and also creates the passive state [altered consciousness] in the meditator to facilitate this fusion of beings.[11] [emphasis added]

The guru generally does not tell the initiate the meaning of the Sanskrit mantra, which are often the names of Hindu gods or proclaim that the self is god. Many mantras include the Sanskrit word 'OM'.

OM (AUM) – The Sound of the Cosmic Motor

Yoga masters vie with each other in proclaiming the grandeur of this syllable. In summary, they teach that OM is the sound of the Cosmic Motor – the sound which Brahman makes in every creative act, so everybody contains that original sound in their memory bank. Its repetition, they claim, invites Brahman and indeed all Hindu gods to enter the mantrist. This invocation of the gods is believed to speed up the process of enlightenment. Its repetition supposedly puts the yogis in touch with the cosmic creation of their minds and facilitates their control of it. Its vibrations create a vacuum in the mind. Hindu scriptures teach that the incarnating ego requires a million years to obtain liberation from maya (illusion). Combined with retarded breathing, the constant use of OM over time is said to be most effective in bringing the yogi to the point of enlightenment, even within the span of one lifetime.

Combined with retarded breathing, it is especially effective in arousing the kundalini.

The word is regarded with deep reverence and awe both in Hindu tradition and in New Age circles, as is exemplified in Vivekananda's lyrical tribute to the invocation when he claims it is by far the most suitable word in any language or in any religion to capture the true nature of God. He, however, seems unaware of the basics of Christianity and would do well to listen to what Peter proclaimed to the Jews after the wondrous outpouring of the Holy Spirit at Pentecost: **'Only in Jesus Christ is there salvation, for of all the names in the world given to humans, this is the only one by which we can be saved.'[12] So for those who are following the way of Jesus Christ as their sole Lord and Saviour, it is the name 'Jesus' which should always be in their hearts and on their lips. The word 'Om', totally unknown in orthodox Christian tradition, should never sully their lips or tarnish their spirit.**

The Guru's blessing

In yoga, a guru traditionally enjoys an exalted and respected position. Having attained enlightenment, the guru, through the ability to enter a trance-like state at will and to work amazing wonders by psychic powers, is acclaimed by disciples as a god and proclaims himself as such. Gurus expect and receive worship from their followers and demand total obedience.

In the rite of initiation, the guru's disciples make a formal act of total surrender accompanied by an act of worship. Gurus respond by giving their blessing which is known as 'the Shakti pat'. Rabi Maharaj defined it as:

> A term used for the touch of a guru, usually of his hand to the worshipper's forehead, that produces supernatural effects. 'Shakti' literally means 'power' and in administering the Shakti pat, the guru becomes a channel of primal power, the cosmic power underlying the universe, embodied in the goddess Shakti, the consort of Shiva.

> The supernatural effect of Shakti through the guru's touch may
> knock the worshipper to the floor, or (s)he may see a bright light
> and receive an experience of enlightenment or inner illumination,
> or have some other mystical or psychic experience.[13]

One of these psychic experiences is commonly the awakening of
the kundalini. In the magazine *Australian Yoga Life*, No 16, an article
entitled 'Growing with the Guru' described the effect of the guru's
blessing on a group of yoga initiates:

> Throughout the year, Swamiji runs retreats that culminate in an
> intensive, a full day of long meditations and talks. At the intensives,
> he imparts formal spiritual initiation in the tradition of his guru,
> called Shaktipat, or the awakening of spiritual energy. He does
> this by touch. This spiritual awakening is also called the kundalini
> awakening. It is based on the ancient path of yoga that describes
> dormant spiritual energy at the base of the spine. When 'awakened',
> this benevolent energy rises within, bringing spiritual insights and
> understanding. Participants at the intensives claim a variety of
> experiences, from seeing inner lights to spiritual revelations or a
> sense of deep peace and contentment.[14]

Nancy Jackson, the author of the article and herself a Swami,
described the awakening of the kundalini as a 'benevolent energy'
resulting in such spiritual delights as 'insights and understanding',
'spiritual revelations', and 'deep peace and contentment'. Others,
however, have experienced another unpredictable and dangerous side
to this 'benevolent energy'.

Sorry, Nobody Home

Since the ultimate purpose of yoga is to lead the adept to experience
that (s)he is one with Brahman, and since Brahman is impersonal, it
follows that the personality of the adept must be destroyed in the
pursuit of enlightenment. And the key to personality is the ego, which

being — suggests — live in the Spirit not the flesh in Christian

includes the intellect, the memory, emotions, desires and the will. All of these have to go, the leading gurus insist.

Two of the key people who sold this 'destruction of the ego' philosophy to the young of the West in the 1970s were Tal Brooke and Ram Dass. Brooke was a member of Sai Baba's inner circle and his key preacher, while Dass, a former Harvard Professor, played a similar role with Muktananda. Tal preached to Western youth flocking to the Baba's ashram in India; Ram crusaded on behalf of Muktananda in America. After 18 months, Brooke saw through Sai Baba, defected, became a Christian and wrote a superb exposé of three power-gurus – Sai Baba, Muktananda and Rajneesh; Dass never lost his faith in Muktananda.

On the subject of 'ego-destruct' Tal Brooke wrote:

> For again, the bottom line was the death of the ego. Something in these [yoga] aspirants had to be destroyed. 'Remember, the you who is the essence of you, is God', Ram Dass had told them. 'That means that your little down-home ethnic American identity is not you – it is your ultimate enemy masquerading as you. So what do you do with this comfortable little ego? You destroy it. With some people it happens fast, with others they hold on and dilly dally.'[15]

One of the most powerful ways of destroying the ego and 'transforming' one's personality is to arouse the kundalini as described here by Ram Dass:

> Kali is an aspect of the Divine Mother, but what a mother to have. She's really gruesome. She scares the hell out of most people. You know why she scares them? Because they want to hold on to who they think they are. She's the fire of purification. She's going to take every single solitary bit of their stash and what will be left are just pure souls floating up into the One … .[16]

But what about the will? In yoga, that is first surrendered to the guru at the point of initiation. Later it is surrendered to the Hindu goddess Kali through the practice of kundalini. And after the so-called state of enlightenment has been reached, it is very difficult to reclaim. Ironically, many of those who go through the process of ego destruction end up with a different personality. Tal Brooke, who ventured some distance along that pathway and has witnessed many others go the full way, claims that the 'new personality' is the result of demonic possession.[17] His detailed studies of the heavy-hitting gurus of the 1970s – Sai Baba, Muktananda and Rajneesh – suggest they have experienced super-possession.[18]

Get a Real Life!

The yoga belief that the only reality in this world is the divine essence in all created things and that whatever is visible, with a beginning and an end, is just a passing mirage, contrasts starkly with God's revelation in the Bible. Christian revelation proudly proclaims not only that all of creation is real but also that after God had completed creation, he 'saw all that he had made, and indeed it was very good'.[19] The pinnacle of God's creation is humanity made 'in the image of God' and given dominion over the whole of creation: 'Be masters of the fish of the sea, the birds of heaven and all the living creatures that move on the earth'.[20] It follows that the human spirit, body and ego are also real and good.

Whereas yoga tends to undervalue the human body and seeks to destroy the ego, Christians rejoice in both and seek to make them docile to the Holy Spirit.

If, as the *Catechism of the Catholic Church* tells us, 'human nature has been wounded in these natural powers proper to it'[21], and that 'the control of the soul's spiritual faculties over the body is shattered'[22], it is also true that with struggle and effort and aided by God's grace, humans can 'succeed in achieving their own inner integrity'.[23] Whereas certain forms of yoga seek to minimise or eliminate the use of the senses, the Christian seeks to nurture and to bring into proper order all the natural faculties: 'Whatever you eat, then, or drink, and whatever else you do, do it all for the glory of God.'[24]

Christian Marriage

The Christian attitude to marriage is also vastly different from that of the yogi. For Christians marriage is:

- essentially good
- a source of holiness for the parents and family
- the core unit of society
- involves serious responsibilities for the parents which cannot be dismissed in the pursuit of a solitary spirituality.

God's revelation bears witness both to the reality of marriage and the commitment of husband and wife to each other.

For this 'communion' to occur, it is essential that man and wife be physically, emotionally and sexually present to each other – 'they become one flesh'. In the normal run of things, they will live together, they will express their mutual love and deepen their communion by sexual intimacy on a regular basis – which requires among other things, physical and emotional presence.

In the Christian understanding of marriage, it is unthinkable that one or both of the couple hive off into a trance-like solitude, or that sexual union be curtailed for extended periods in the pursuit of kundalini as was the case with Rabi Maharaj's parents. And it would be a serious neglect of one's responsibilities towards one's spouse and children if one opted for yogic solitude. What St John Baptist de la Salle says to teachers is relevant also to parents involved in the hurly burly of raising a family today:

> Do not make the slightest distinction between the duties of your state and what pertains to your salvation and perfection. Rest

assured that you will never effect your salvation more certainly and that you will never acquire greater perfection than by fulfilling well the duties of your state, provided you do so with a view to accomplishing the will of God.[25]

4

Monkeying with Minds in the Monastery

Yoga has made significant entries into the Catholic Church. One movement was centred in India and the other in France, occurring almost simultaneously in the mid-1950s. In the East, the famous, controversial priest Bede Griffiths sought to combine Hindu yoga with Christianity, while in France Jean-Marie Déchanet sought to divorce yoga from its Hindu roots and establish a purely Christian variety.[1] Both priests had a background in monasticism.

Griffiths had been an English Benedictine, left the congregation shortly after arriving in India and remained a priest until the last few years of his life, when he established his ashramic and yogic monks as part of the Camaldolese-Benedictines. This, he hoped, would ensure their continuity once he died.

And then in more recent years, three eminent spiritual writers, all American Trappist monks, have had a powerful influence on the Catholic Church in the West through their practice of mind-altering techniques – Thomas Merton, Thomas Keating and Basil Pennington.

Into India

In 1956 Bede set out for India where he established a Christian ashram in association with a Cistercian monk in Kerala. Their aim was to establish a monastery within the ashram. The Cistercian was the Prior and Bede the Sub-Prior. After 10 years they had achieved their goal, with their monastic ashram housing about 20 monks. However, tensions between the Prior and Sub-Prior grew to a point of crisis, as the Prior, with some justification, felt that Bede was undermining his authority. As a result, Bede left to establish his own monastic ashram in Tamil Nadu, seeking to combine the Benedictine and Hindu traditions.

From the moment of his arrival in India, Bede took to the Indian culture and the Hindu religion like a duck to water. For the rest of his life he was to steep himself in the study of the Hindu scriptures and the practice of yoga, and it was not long before he was referring to himself as a 'Christian Yogi'. By the time he established his second ashram, called 'Shantivanam', he enjoyed a great degree of latitude, for being the authority figure in the ashram he was not constrained by higher superiors. He made sure that the ashram was independent of the local Church. Bede and the young men who joined his community practised yoga and adopted the garb of Hindu yogis.[2]

In the years following, he wrote a number of articles about yoga, but not a great deal about his own personal experience of it. However, there is a glimpse of the effects the practice of kundalini yoga was having on his personal life in a passage of a letter he wrote to a friend, which his biographer attests referred to the power of kundalini:

> India has released in me the forces of the unconscious, which were previously submerged, and I have sometimes been terrified to find the demonic power which is within me. This is the 'dragon' as you say, which is in all of us. The spiritual life consists in the conversion of this power. We cannot destroy it or suppress it. It is not evil in itself, it is a holy power (as the Hindu genius has so well discovered).[3]

It is interesting that, in the same breath, Bede describes kundalini arousal as both a metaphoric 'demonic' and a 'holy' power. But there is no doubt from the text that this form of yoga has his wholehearted endorsement.

Elsewhere in his writings Bede makes it clear that he wholeheartedly approved of kundalini and raja yoga:

> This is the goal of Christian yoga, body and soul are to be transfigured by the divine life and to participate in the divine consciousness. There is descent of the Spirit into matter and a corresponding ascent, by which matter is transformed by the indwelling power of the Spirit and the body is transfigured. In kundalini yoga this is represented as the union of Shiva and Shakti in the human body. The divine power is represented as coiled up like a serpent at the base of the spine. This divine energy has to be led through the seven chakras, or centres of psychic energy, until it reaches the thousand petalled lotus at the crown of the head. Then Shiva, who is pure consciousness, unites with Shakti, the divine energy in nature, and body and soul are transformed. This is very different from the [raja] yoga of Patanjali... Yet both these yogas have their place.[4]

In the same article Bede revealed: 'Wisdom consists of the knowledge of being in pure consciousness without any modification, and this brings lasting bliss.'[5]

This 'yogaspeak' means that true wisdom consists in creating a vacuum in the mind so that all thought ceases. At that point, self-realisation occurs, accompanied by feelings of bliss.

Bede's Hybrid Yoga

Throughout his life, Bede maintained that the practice of yoga could be a great help in leading a Christian life, particularly in leading a deeply contemplative prayer life. He rejected pantheism and viewed the human as being immersed in God, but not of the same essence as God. He equated the Brahman of Hinduism with the Holy Spirit of Christianity. And he sought to incarnate his yogic prayer in everyday life by following the 'integral philosophy' of Sri Aurobindo. As a yogic mantra, he sometimes used – 'Jesus son of David have mercy on me'.

Though Bede referred to himself as a Christian yogi, his yoga was basically Hindu yoga, elements of which were dressed up in Christian terms. Yet such yoga could easily undermine the faith of a true Christian.

Bede had no problem accepting the psychic powers which accompany yoga. He naively sees these occult powers as being common to the shamans of pagan religions and the prophets of the Judeo-Christian religion: 'Not only shamans but all the prophets, seers and visionaries of the past were people who had these psychic powers and psychic vision. The method is to open ourselves through intuition to these deeper insights and then try to understand them and appropriately to systematise them through reason.'[6]

If Bede's teaching on spirituality was unsound, his judgment on yoga-related practices was more disturbing. One of Bede's obvious blind spots was his exaltation, in true Hindu fashion, of the mantra 'OM'. Before reading the Vedas, he was accustomed to recite the Gayatri mantra (which is preceded by 'OM') three times. 'It [OM] is a sacred word', Bede related in a masterly piece of understatement 'like Amen from the Hebrew.'[7] He knew well that 'OM' is the highest form of praise one can give to Brahman and the other Hindu gods. It is also the most powerful way of invoking their presence within one.

Such importance did this mantra have for Bede and members of his Shantivanam community that they established the cosmic cross with OM at the centre, as their official symbol, erected in the grounds of the Shantivanam ashram. It has a Sanskrit OM in the centre and the congregation's motto in Sanskrit written on it, the meaning of which is: *We try to live our Benedictine life in the context of Indian spirituality, that is in the recognition of the Divine Presence in the whole cosmos and in the centre of our own being.*[8]

Members of the congregation wear a small version of this cross around their necks, with the motto being sufficiently ambiguous as to be acceptable to some Hindus and Christians. One is left wondering what part the unique Lordship of Jesus Christ plays in this Benedictine community.

Meditating with Maharishi

Bede's singular lack of discernment was also evident in the unqualified endorsement he gave the Transcendental Movement of Maharishi Mahesh Yogi. This form of meditation was plucked straight out of Hindu yoga, transported to the West as a 'scientific technique for relaxation,'[9] and marketed as non-religious Transcendental Meditation or TM.

What made it so marketable to a generation starved of religious experience was its utter simplicity. All that was required was the recitation of a mantra for 20 minutes, morning and evening. This, purportedly, would lead to numerous benefits ranging from a stress-free existence to a high level of creativity. Asked what he thought of TM, Bede replied: *It is to me completely convincing. It seems to me to be a method that is physiologically and spiritually sound... there is nothing in [this] theory of states of consciousness which a Catholic could not accept.*[10]

Not all Christians shared Bede's naïve optimism.

The Initiation Rite

Despite the constant claim of TM promoters that this form of meditation is purely secular, a close analysis of the initiation ceremony reveals that TM is steeped deeply in the Hindu Vedantic tradition. Vail Hamilton, a former TM teacher provides an insight into the true nature of the rite which she conducted with many initiates:

> At the beginning of the ceremony the candidate is asked to bring an offering of six flowers, three pieces of fresh fruit, and a white handkerchief, which are placed on an altar before a picture of Guru Dev (which means 'Divine Leader'), who is the Maharishi's departed Master. The small room is candlelit and filled with incense.

The candidate is asked to stand before this altar while the teacher sings a hymn [puja] of thanksgiving and praise to the entire line of departed Hindu masters who have passed down the knowledge of the mantras. At the end of the song, the teacher indicates to the person that (s)he is to kneel for a few moments of silence, and then, both still kneeling, the teacher repeats the mantra selected for the person and has her/him repeat it until s(he) has correctly pronounced it, and then they are seated for further instruction.

Many candidates I encountered while teaching TM objected to this religious aspect, but went along with it in order to learn the technique. Once they experienced the pleasant sensation of meditating, they quickly forgot their immediate objection to the religious nature of the ceremony and rapidly embraced all that TM had to offer them.[11]

In the Hindu tradition, a super-guru such as Guru Dev, is commonly worshipped by his disciples, particularly during the process of initiation. The following are all part of the act of worship in this ceremony:

• offering of personal gifts to Guru Dev
• lit candles and incense
• standing in front of Guru Dev's picture while the hymn is being sung
• silent kneeling in front of Guru Dev's picture.

Candidates who expressed concern about the religious aspect of this rite would be even more concerned if they understood the language (sanskrit) of the hymn and of the mantra. In part, the hymn translates as: 'To Lord Narayana, to lotus-born Brahma, the Creator... to Shankaracharya the redeemer, hailed as Krishna... I bow down. To the glory of the Lord I bow down again and again, at whose door the whole galaxy of gods pray for perfection day and night. Adorned with immeasurable glory, preceptor of the whole world, having bowed down to him, we gain fulfilment.'[12]

Often unbeknown, candidates are caught up in the worship of a pantheon of Hindu gods! Candidates also have to learn the mantra, allegedly a meaningless syllable.[13] However, 'recent research has revealed ... that far from being 'meaningless sounds', TM mantras are inseparably related to the names of Hindu deities.[14]

Because the mantras are also in the sacred Hindu language of Sanskrit, unsuspecting initiates have no idea that they are invoking a Hindu deity.

Cardinal Sin Speaks Out

In 1984, Cardinal Sin, then Catholic Archbishop of Manila, presented his flock with a blistering doctrinal critique of Maharishi's teaching and technique:[15]

- Maharishi's 'god' is impersonal as opposed to the God of Christian Revelation, a personal God who loves each human person in an intimate way.
- By preaching that 'All is one', Mahariji offers a form of pantheism.
- Through TM, man is considered capable of attaining unlimited perfection, of being totally liberated from all pain and suffering.
- Maharishi's approach to the problem of pain and suffering implies the rejection of the redemptive value of suffering and of the existence of Christ as the Redeemer.
- Maharishi tries to ignore the existence of sin.

Cardinal Sin argued: 'One cannot be a Christian and a Maharishi.'

TM and Demonic Influence

One of the real dangers for adepts of TM is that it makes people quite vulnerable to negative spiritual influences. After practising yoga, Mary, profiled earlier, graduated to TM. After two years practice she began to experience feelings of lesbianism, the result of which was a sexual reversal:

> I noticed that while in deep meditation periods the white light that we always sought seemed to be getting darker and noisier. And at work my feelings for one particular work mate, the one whose face appeared to me at night, were getting, can I say, unhealthy. I thought: what is happening here? I am a married woman with a loving husband and family. My whole sexual identity seemed to have turned upside down. I found myself admiring beautiful women instead of handsome men.[16]

After renouncing her involvement in TM and returning to the practice of her Catholic faith, Mary's homosexual feelings faded. She has since enjoyed a happy married life.

Vail, a former TM teacher, who moved into a more advanced level of TM, while doing a teacher training course in Italy in 1972, also came under what seemed to be a strong demonic influence. She relates: 'One night I awoke with a sense of fear because a spirit was putting pressure all over my body and head in an attempt to enter my body. I commanded it to leave and resisted until it left. Other supernatural experiences also began to occur – ESP and clairvoyance, telepathy and the beginnings of astral travel.'[17]

In terms of spiritual development through the technique of TM, Bede would have done well to have given serious consideration to the then-Cardinal Ratzinger's wise words about Christian mysticism, directed to Christians who were practising yoga, Zen meditation and TM:

> Without a doubt, a Christian needs certain periods of retreat into solitude to be recollected and, in God's presence, rediscover his path. Nevertheless, given his character as a creature, and a creature who knows that only in grace is he secure, his method of drawing closer to God is not based on any 'technique' in the strict sense of the word. That would contradict the spirit of childhood called for by the gospel. Genuine Christian mysticism has nothing to do with technique: it is always a gift of God, and the one who benefits from it knows himself to be unworthy.[18]

Cardinal Ratzinger's warning takes on added significance in light of the reality that the technique of TM so highly recommended by Bede, was clearly occultic.

Zen and a Monk Called Merton

As a postscript, it is worth including a very brief treatment of Thomas Merton's involvement in Zen meditation. Many Christians have justified their involvement in New Age activities by reference to Merton's involvement in Zen, Dumoulin's description of which is succinct and accurate: 'Zen ... is the name of a Mahayana Buddhist school of meditation originating in China and characterised by the practice of meditation in the lotus position (Japanese, zazen) and the use of the koan, as well as by the enlightenment experience of satori.'[19]

At the heart of Zen is meditation. As in yoga, this is characterised by controlled breathing and the focusing of the mind on one 'point' – in this case one's breathing. The purpose of both the controlled breathing and the point-focus is the same as in raja yoga – to progressively eliminate all thoughts. The ultimate in this mind control is the creation of a complete void. When the adept reaches that point, one experiences a state of utter bliss and a sense of oneness with the cosmos. This experience of Ultimate Reality is termed 'Nirvana'.

The other Zen technique used for creating a void in the mind is the koan, the purpose of which is to 'disrupt the sequence of logical thought and so bring about enlightenment by inducing an altered state of consciousness'.[20]

Zen Comes to Merton

By the late 1950s, the most famous monk living in a Cistercian monastery buried in the woodhills of Kentucky was undoubtedly Thomas Merton. A prolific author, he had written a number of impressive works on spirituality to the point where his name had become a by-word among Catholics. In the last decade of his life, he showed an interest in Eastern religions and spiritualities. Possibly due to his influence, the representatives of a variety of spiritual traditions were invited to display their wares to the monks at 'Gethsemani', their monastery. In his book *Mystics and Zen Masters*, published in 1961, Merton proclaims:

> Within the last two or three years, the Abbey of Gethsemani has been visited by men experienced and fully qualified to represent such traditions as Raja Yoga, Zen, Hasidism, Tibetan Buddhism, Sufism, etc. The names of these would be instantly recognised as among the most distinguished in their field. Therefore, the question of contacts and actual communication between contemplatives of the various traditions no longer presents very great obstacles. A little experience of such dialogue shows at once that this is precisely the most fruitful and most rewarding of ecumenical exchange.[21]

It would seem that the monks of Gethsemani were anticipating by some seven years, the type of dialogue encouraged by Vatican II: *The Church therefore urges her sons to enter with prudence and charity into discussion and collaboration with members of other [non-Christian] religions.*[22]

With more haste than the prudence recommended by the Council, Merton moved from dialogue to action. He took up the practice of Zen meditation with a view to enriching his own Christian prayer life and bringing about renewal in his monastic living.

In going down the path of Zen, Merton sought to divorce the meditation techniques from its Buddhist tradition, bringing to the lotus pose his own Christian tradition. His guide in this was the world renowned authority, D.T. Suzuki, whose books Merton read avidly and with whom he kept in regular correspondence, even meeting with him personally on one occasion.

After some experience of this Eastern discipline, Merton came to the conviction that '[Zen] can shine through this or that system, religious or irreligious, just as light can shine through glass that is blue, green, or red or yellow.'[23]

One is left wondering where faith in Christ fits into the whole framework of Zen. It appears, in Merton's opinion, to be a technique which operates automatically and independently of faith. And yet in the view of his biographer, William Shannon, Merton was convinced that for him, Zen was a form of Christian contemplation.[24]

In late 1977, Marilyn Ferguson, the high priestess of the New Age movement at that time wrote a best-selling book *The Aquarian Conspiracy* mentioning that she sent a questionnaire to 210 persons who were actively committed to spreading the New Age message. The great majority were resident in the USA. One hundred and eighty-five responded to the survey.

The responses to one particular question are of interest: 'When respondents were asked to name individuals whose ideas had influenced them either through personal contact or through their writings, those most often named in order of frequency were Pierre Teilhard de Chardin, C.G. Jung,[25] Abraham Maslow, Carl Rogers, Aldous Huxley, Roberto Assagioli and J. Krishnamurti.

'Others frequently mentioned were: Paul Tillich, Hermann Hesse,[26]Alfred North Whitehead, Martin Buber, Ruth Benedict, Margaret Mead, Gregory Bateson, Tarthaug Tulku, Alan Watts, Sri Aurobindo,[27] Swami Muktananda, D.T. Suzuki, Thomas Merton ...[28].

This list is also quoted in the Vatican document, *Jesus Christ the Bearer of the Water of Life, A Christian reflection on the 'New Age,'* which makes it clear that New Age belief and practice are incompatible with orthodox Christianity. Thomas Merton in his later practice and teaching associated with Zen, like a Pied Piper, is with others, leading people down the slippery slope of New Age, and one of those on whom he had a profound influence was his fellow Trappist and good friend, Basil Pennington.

Fatal Flaws

One of Merton's major errors was to confuse a mind-emptying, human technique with Christian contemplation, which is always a grace of

God. Addressing such confusion, the then Cardinal Ratzinger, as Prefect of the Congregation for the Doctrine of the Faith, issued a letter to all Catholic Bishops, *On Some Aspects of Christian Meditation.*

The letter provided guidelines for Christians seeking to fuse 'Zen, Transcendental Meditation or Yoga' with Christian prayer. There are two statements in it which are particularly relevant to Merton's situation: 'Still others [Christians] do not hesitate to place that absolute without images or concepts which is proper to Buddhist theory, on the same level as the majesty of God revealed in Christ, which towers above finite reality.'[29]

The document quotes John Paul II: '... the call of Teresa of Jesus advocating a prayer completely centred on Christ is valid even in our day, against some methods of prayer which are not inspired by the Gospel and which in practice tend to set Christ aside in preference for a mental void which makes no sense in Christianity.'[30]

As well as Zen's incompatibility with Christian prayer, another vital factor to be considered is that techniques designed to alter the state of consciousness and create a void in the mind open the practitioner to the danger of demonic influence. It is for good reason that Basilea Schlink, an astute observer, gives a stern warning about yoga and Zen: 'With regard to yoga, a Christian today can only choose between Christ and Belial [Satan], for the possibility of combining yoga with the Christian faith does not exist. (The same applies to Zen, the corresponding Japanese teaching which stems from Buddhism, and is likewise spreading in the West).'[31]

Centring Prayer – Pseudo Contemplation

In response to a challenge to the Trappist monks from Pope Paul VI to encourage the contemplative dimension in the Catholic Church at large, Father Thomas Keating, Abbot of St Joseph's Monastery in Massachusetts, together with his monks, began to hold dialogue with Hindu and Buddhist representatives. The upshot was that an ex-Trappist monk conducted a session of TM for the monks, and a Zen Master for the next eight years conducted two 7-day retreats annually which the Abbot and a significant number of monks attended.[32]

During this period of the 70s, Keating and Father Basil Pennington, the Professor of Spirituality in the monastery, sought to fuse elements of the TM technique with the Catholic contemplative tradition, which approach (under the influence of Thomas Merton) has come to be known as Centring Prayer (C.P.) This quickly mushroomed into a world-wide movement which has created a climate of opinion amongst many Christians that the technique of voiding the mind can provide a short-cut to infused contemplative prayer and inner healing.

C.P. is promoted as a technique which leads one to the direct experience of God in contemplative prayer. Like TM, it is practised for 20 minutes morning and evening. And like T.M. it involves the repetition of a sacred word which for all intents and purposes has the same effect as a mantra, its effect being to remove all thoughts and feeling from the mind as Keating informs us: 'As you go down deeper, you reach a place where the sacred word disappears altogether and there are no thoughts. This is often experienced as a suspension of consciousness, a space.'[33]

This altered state of consciousness [A.S.C.] purportedly brings one automatically into contact with the True Self which is allegedly God: '…God and our True Self are the same thing'.[34] Through the regular practice of C.P., one comes to realise one's own divinity as in T.M. as we hear on one of Keating's video introductions: 'Listen as Father Thomas offers you the invitation to become God.'[35] This experience of self-realisation is allegedly accompanied by the evacuation of negative emotions characteristic of the False Self.

Pennington claims that C.P. is 'a new name for an ancient form of prayer'[36], and in C.P. teaching, classic prayer authorities often invoked to substantiate this claim are John Cassian, the anonymous author of

The Cloud of Unknowing, and St Teresa of Avila. A study of each of these writers makes it clear that Keating and Pennington have sorely misinterpreted them.

Cassian, for example, addressing beginners in the life of prayer, recommends the repetition of a single psalm verse, 'O God come to my aid, O Lord make haste to help me.'[37] The novice in prayer takes this as the sole topic for his meditations; the continual repetition of this aspiration throughout the day 'keeps the **mind** wholly and entirely upon God…[this verse] carries within it all the **feelings** of which human nature is capable'[38] (emphasis added). Over time, the aspiration and its meaning become a part of one's personality. In this process, the mind and feelings are fully engaged and at no point does the mind become a void.

Unlike Cassian, the author of *The Cloud* directs his advice to one who had advanced to the initial stages of infused contemplation and in treating of such he makes it patently clear that 'techniques and methods are ultimately useless for awakening contemplative love.'[39]

In her comprehensive teaching St Teresa of Avila covers all stages of the spiritual life. For beginners, she recommends discursive forms of prayer which should bear fruit in the practice of the Christian virtues. This she considers the best foundation for contemplative prayer. However, she hastens to warn that 'however diligent our efforts we cannot acquire it … It is given only to whom God wills to give it and often when the soul is least thinking of it.'[40]

And she issues a strong warning to those who would seek to empty the mind of all thought: 'If His Majesty has not begun to absorb us [in contemplative prayer], I cannot understand how the mind can be stopped. There's no way of doing so without bringing more harm than good … However, once God graces the person with the gift of infused prayer, the intellect ceases to work because **God suspends it. Taking it upon oneself to stop and suspend thought is what I mean should not be done; nor should we cease to work with the**

**intellect, because otherwise we would be left like cold simpletons
and be doing neither one thing nor the other**[41] (emphasis added).

To give the impression that C.P. is but a new name for traditional
forms of contemplative prayer in the Church is both untrue and
quite misleading. And current Church teaching indicates that C.P.
is neither Christian nor prayer. The then-Cardinal Ratzinger in his
watershed document on Christian meditation, quotes John Paul II
who maintained that creating a mental void in prayer 'has no place in
Christianity.'[42] The *Catechism* (2726) echoes this view, stating that 'the
effort of concentration to reach a mental void' is an erroneous notion
of prayer.

That C.P. may result in the spiritually and psychologically dangerous
state of an A.S.C. is verified by observation. Keating relates that
in the early days of the C.P. workshops in the monastery, some of
the monks and guests 'complained that it was spooky seeing people
walking around the guest-house like zombies.'[43] Commenting on this,
Father Dreher drily remarks: 'They recognised the symptoms but
could not diagnose the illness.'[44]

One of Keating's disciples commented to him that he was having
a hard time coming out of an altered state of consciousness during
Mass and could not concentrate. Keating fully endorsed his situation
by telling him: 'That is a nice problem to have.'[45]

Fr. Dreher received a letter from the mother of a 10-year-old girl
who had been taught C.P. in her religion classes by a Catholic religious
Sister for a period of two-and-a-half years. The mother wrote:

> About six weeks ago, Kristy started having difficulty going to
> sleep. She didn't want to stay in her own room and would lie there
> afraid to close her eyes until I would let her go into her sister's
> room and sleep with her. Finally she confided in me that she could
> see something scary if she closed her eyes. A few days ago she
> confided that it laughed. Kristy had used the C.P. on her own at
> bedtime for some time before this started.[46]

Fr. Dreher suspects that Kristy's practice of C.P. may have 'opened her to evil spirits and such harassments.'[47]

What is of equal concern is the serious lack of discernment which both Keating and Pennington show towards various New Age mind-altering practices which have a high compatibility with C.P. Pennington is an ardent advocate of TM,[48] while Keating encourages his disciples to do yoga[49] and tai chi,[50] and is so supportive of kundalini yoga that he wrote a foreword endorsing the practice in a book written on the topic in which he states that 'Kundalini is an enormous energy for good'[51] and that '... this energy can arise through the practice of ordinary Christian prayer forms ...'.[52]

Sadly, not only have two high-profile leaders in the Catholic Church created a pseudo contemplation but they have also encouraged many Christians to embrace Hindu, Buddhist and Taoist practices which have more in common with New Age[53] than with orthodox Christianity.

5

A Genuine Christian
Alternative to Yoga

As this book was about to be published, I was given a DVD[1] with an accompanying booklet[2] called *Praise Moves*. The description on the cover says: 'A Christian Alternative to Yoga.' I was most impressed by the programme and its presentation. Its author and presenter, Laurette Willis, is described on the DVD cover as a Womens' Fitness Specialist and a certified personal trainer. In her article, 'Why a Christian Alternative to Yoga' which appears on her *Praise Moves* website, she provides some background:

> As a child growing up in Long Island, I became involved in yoga at the age of seven when my mother and I began watching a daily yoga exercise programme on television. For the next 22 years I was heavily involved with yoga, metaphysics and the New Age Movement until I came to the end of myself and surrendered my life to Jesus Christ in 1987.[3]

After becoming a Christian, she abandoned her New Age practices including yoga. But 14 years later, the Spirit of God moved her in a new direction:

> I was looking for a gentler form of exercise. I'd been doing aerobics, and I wanted to do some stretching and strengthening exercises, but I wanted absolutely nothing to do with yoga. I wondered how I might exercise the body while praising God, how I might meditate on scripture while stretching the body – moving

in praise to God. Praising and moving – Praise Moves!... For the
next two years I prayed, studied and developed the Praise-Moves
series of stretching postures. I wanted to make sure this was not
just a good idea but God's idea.[4]

By 2006, Laurette was in a position to produce her alternative to
yoga for Christians, which she stresses, is not Christian yoga, which
she sees as a contradiction in terms. At the heart of her *Praise Moves*
is a set of 21 postures, each animated by a passage of Scripture. For
example, The Eagle posture is accompanied by the speaking aloud of
this verse: 'Those who wait upon the Lord shall renew their strength;
they shall mount up with wings as eagles, they shall run and not be
weary, they shall walk and not faint' (Is 40:31).[5]

Praise Moves is designed for committed Christians. Its foundation
text makes that eminently clear: 'For you were brought at a price;
therefore glorify God in your body and in your spirit which are God's'
(1Cor 6:20).

Through this process, Laurette claims and users testify, one can
obtain all the health and relaxation benefits attributed to yoga.

One can do this programme in the comfort of one's home by doing
it in synch with the DVD or as part of a class under the guidance of
one of Laurette's many qualified instructors. Such is the popularity of
the course, that it is now available throughout America and has been
introduced to a number of countries world-wide. A correspondence
course is being offered to train instructors in Australia.

Laurette has also developed a fitness programme for children,
Power Moves Kids. It combines stretching exercises with character-
building quotes. It is non-religious and is being used in schools both
public and private. See the website, **http://praisemoves.com**.

Part B

TAI CHI

6

Just an Innocent Pastime

In Australia today, tai chi like yoga is big business and is seen by the health profession and the populace as a means to good health, physical and emotional. Even the martial art form, tai chi chuan (boxing), is regarded as the gentlest of the martial arts, lacking the aggression which some find disconcerting in the hard martial arts. To consider tai chi in any way harmful, is generally regarded as erroneous and alarmist.

Tai chi is commonly marketed as a means of:

- reducing stress
- improving physical and emotional health
- self-defence in the form of a martial art
- fostering spiritual development.

Tai chi comprises:

- gentle, balanced relaxation exercises
- slow, rhythmic, abdominal breathing
- forms of meditation:

    focusing on one's breathing

    visualising one's movements

    visualising the movement of chi within the body

    feeling the chi move.

The purpose of this 'meditation in movement' is to:

- empty the mind
- produce an altered state of consciousness.

73

Chi stored just below the navel:

- can give incredible strength in combat
- may be used to heal oneself and others.

Chi Kung

Chi kung (Qigong), is a first cousin of tai chi. Whereas tai chi is physically active, chi kung is physically passive. In chi kung, one takes up a yoga-like posture, remaining completely still. Breathing, as in yoga, is controlled and retarded. The methods of meditation are similar to those used in raja yoga/ zen meditation. The purpose of meditation, as in yoga, is to:

- empty the mind
- alter the state of consciousness.

Retarded breathing and meditation as in tai chi, result in:

- cultivation
- storage
- movement of chi within the body.

Ominously, however, the ultimate achievement in tai chi as in chi kung is to become divine. Chi may also be used like prana to rouse the kundalini. This commonly results in the experience of a range of occult powers.

Channelling the Chi

According to Chinese medical theory, chi is transmitted throughout the body along a series of energy channels called meridians. There are 14 such channels. It is from major energy centres that chi radiates out via the meridians to every cell in the body. By far the most significant of these is that situated just below the navel. It is commonly referred to in tai chi circles as the tan tien. This term means literally 'field of breath',[1] or expressed more popularly, 'sea of chi'.[2]

Authorities differ as to the number of major energy centres. Kenneth Cohen, noted American chi kung scholar and practitioner lists three:

1. The lower tan tien [the tan tien], 3-7cm below the navel.

2. The middle tan tien at the level of the heart

3. The upper tan tien between the eyebrows [the third eye].[3]

Whenever the term tan tien is used in tai chi/chi kung, it generally refers to the lower tan tien.

In a healthy person, according to the philosophy of tai chi, chi flows harmoniously in good ying-yang balance to all parts of the body. However, most people have blockages to the flow of chi in different parts of the body. Tai chi, it is claimed, provides a remedy to such blockages: As the Tai Chi exercises release tension from various parts of the body, the channels are re-opened and the flow of chi is re-established.[4]

Proficiency in the ability to control the flow of chi provides the adept with a range of psychic gifts, the most prominent being superhuman powers of strength and ability to heal oneself and others.

In researching this book, I interviewed Elizabeth. Now of mature years, she struck me as having a solid Christian spirituality and gave me the impression that she has both feet planted firmly on the ground. In the course of the interview, she related this story:

> What did I know of tai chi? Absolutely nothing, except what I had learned from observing senior citizens in garden settings. Watching these, I had formed the idea that tai chi was a series of exercises done at a somewhat slowly controlled speed. It didn't appear difficult and I wondered about its value as a form of exercise.
>
> One day in a shopping mall in Canberra I happened upon a tai chi demonstration. I went to watch. What I witnessed there in the mall was very different from what I had observed in a variety

of park areas. Movements were controlled, but where those previously witnessed were fluid, these were stronger, much more aggressive and quicker. They were more the style I would have expected of a kung-fu performer and I felt very apprehensive watching the young man performing. He was in battle mode and there was no mistaking it. He also appeared to be seeking out a target. Such was my apprehension I moved away from the area but as I moved I noticed the young man's movements were following me. To break further contact, I moved into a shoe-shop only to be followed there by a powerful psychic force. What happened next frightened me and certainly startled the shop assistant. I was literally attacked even at that distance by whatever power emanated from that young man and I felt the impact in my back through to my chest. Such was the violence of the attack I lost balance and the shocked assistant helped me into a chair. She had no idea what had happened, though she could see whatever it was had left me feeling decidedly unwell.

At this stage I did not know that tai chi was also a martial art. It was not until months later that I learned this and had no trouble believing it as I had suffered a wounding already. Ever since this experience many years ago, I have been disturbed to find so many people involved in tai chi, particularly as I have noticed that those who practise it become more aggressive and tend to strike out in a variety of ways at other people.

Before the sceptical reader writes this off as hysteria, let me recount a much more public and dramatic account of the same phenomenon seen by millions on American television:

> In the award–winning, nationally televised 1993 PBS series *Healing and the Mind*, host Bill Moyers discussed the popularity of the martial arts and the amazing powers they offer. In one segment, both Moyers and the martial arts students were astounded as a 90-year-old tai chi master used the mystical energy called chi to send an entire line of adepts tumbling to the ground by merely

throwing chi at them from a distance of some six metres. Interviews with the students afterwards revealed they felt forced down by a mysterious and irresistible power. This was the power they themselves were seeking, although they were warned it would take many years of austere discipline to acquire.[5]

Such dramatic examples of the power of chi are not rare in the realms of tai chi as a martial art. But it is not from this perspective that tai chi is generally marketed in Australia.

Christians Welcome the Chi

The Lidcombe Catholic Club tells us that 'The art of Tai Chi stimulates physical and mental well-being amongst practitioners. Gentle stretching and specific Tai Chi movements assist with circulation and muscular toning, while relaxing the mind at the same time.'[6] This kind of spiel, common nowadays in clubs, gyms and retirement homes, presents tai chi as the most innocent and healthy of pastimes.

The spread of tai chi is in no way limited to the secular world. In researching this book, I approached a senior member of a Chinese Christian Church near Liverpool. This elderly Chinese man lived only three doors away from me, and I used to see him entering his house in a van with the name of his church on it. Since the man was both Chinese and Christian, I thought he might be able to give me some interesting insights into tai chi. What was my surprise when he opened the door, and I found him dressed in a white tai-chi uniform. He was an instructor of tai chi in his local church, and one point he made, mainly by sign language, was that tai chi was very good for the heart and for the circulation. It brought home to me how enthusiastically this meditation in movement was being embraced by Christians.

Participants at some Catholic retreat/renewal centres, for example, may avail themselves of the opportunity of rising early to separate the clouds and embrace the chi-filled sun in tai chi classes. As well as centring on the chi-within or the Holy Spirit – take your pick – this group activity is sometimes touted as a means of promoting unity among the retreatants, despite the fact that some may be less than happy to march with The Force.

One retreat centre in NSW provides an explanatory sheet on tai chi, promoting a local academy. The sheet makes no mention of the dangerous philosophy on which tai chi is based. Perhaps the keen interest in tai chi in Catholic spirituality centres might account for the enthusiasm of so many religious Sisters for tai chi. As the young man behind the counter at one tai chi shop told me, *Even Catholic Sisters, once they realise that tai chi is not a religion but a philosophy, they get really enthusiastic about it!*

With the promotion elements in the Catholic Church are giving tai chi, I suspect a good number of religious houses in Australia have a copy of one of the popular videos on the subject.

Tai chi has also progressed from spirituality centres to Catholic schools. In one diocese in NSW, it is not uncommon for school staff to participate in a session of tai chi as part of a staff spirituality day, with the backing of the Catholic Education Office, as I discovered when I questioned the practice. One cannot help wondering if the next logical step will be to introduce tai chi or a modified version under another name into physical education programmes in schools. Should any concerned parents raise objections on religious grounds, they would be politely but firmly informed, as I was, that tai chi is completely neutral. It is based on philosophy and has nothing to do with religion.

So what's the Problem?

Tai chi teachers are correct when they proclaim that tai chi is based on the philosophy of Taoism and not on the religion of Taoism which developed some 500 years after the philosophy. **But what many** fail to realise is that the Taoist philosophy is itself a system of religious beliefs.

My thesis is:

1. **Tai chi, imported from China, is inextricably linked with a system of religious beliefs called Taoist philosophy.**
2. **The key beliefs of Taoist philosophy clash head-on with the beliefs of Christianity.**
3. **Altering one's state of consciousness, a practice common to tai chi and chi kung, is highly dangerous spiritually. It can easily open one up to demonic influences and may result in occult powers, a number of which are specifically condemned in the Bible.**

Meditation in Movement

Hundreds of thousands of Australians have learned tai chi, in person or working through the movements with the help of DVDs. Ideally, the slow, graceful movements have some resonance with nature and are:

- slow and quiet
- harmonious
- free-flowing and continuous.

Beyond the physical, however, the place of the mind is important in each movement. One of the chief aims of tai chi is to create a balance between the mind and the body. This begins even before one begins the movements by doing some mindful breathing, focusing the mind on slow, rhythmic, abdominal breathing.

During the exercises, the mind leads the movement by imaging it. For example, when the practitioner is doing the rowing the boat movement, the mind visualises the body in its action of rowing a boat, and watches the body doing so. In this way, the mind and the body are brought into harmony. Ideally, this keeps the mind in present time throughout the session, focused solely on the bodily movements. The effect is to progressively lessen the stream of consciousness, inducing a sense of deep relaxation and an altered state of consciousness.

In Taoist philosophy, the process is referred to as *emptying the mind*.[7] It is believed that at the point of emptiness, the unconscious mind becomes highly receptive to cosmic chi.

Tai chi is geared to bring about the cultivation, movement and storage of chi. The balancing of body parts in each movement allegedly produces chi and causes it to flow through the body; and the balancing of mind-body produces the same results. Participants are encouraged to visualise and feel the flow of chi in different parts of the body.

As the sessions end, participants are guided to place both hands gently on the stomach and to breathe abdominally for a few minutes, resulting in the storage of chi just below the navel.

Masterly Marketing

Tai chi has faced two hurdles in Australia. The first was to gain acceptance for such a *gentle, non-physical art from such a sporting nation*.[8] The second was to gain similar acceptance in a Western country possessed of a significant number of Christians or of people with a Christian background, many of whom would be inclined to look with suspicion on any spiritual art form emerging out of *pagan China*. But with a passion born of tai chi, its masters have set to work with determination and an innate shrewdness. Conscious that many Australians in the 1980s were stressing out; that the Western world was becoming increasingly pre-occupied with health and longevity, its promoters honed in on these areas.

Using shrewdness and diplomacy, it was successfully marketed to those with Christian backgrounds with a muted version of Taoist philosophy. Proponents claim that the philosophy of Taoism is not a religion, but overlook the fact that it is a system of religious beliefs. Tai chi's proponents insist that Taoism makes no judgement as to whether the Tao was uncreated. **But the *bible* of Taoist philosophy, the *Tao Te Ching*, makes it unambiguously clear that the Tao is uncreated – it is eternal,[9] which means it has no beginning, it always was**.

While presenting chi as *intrinsic energy* or *life-force*, not as a divine force, proponents and teachers often fail to mention the underlying philosophy that all created things are divine manifestations of chi and that the ultimate purpose of tai chi is to enable the practitioner to become divine.

Such a muted presentation of the philosophy behind tai chi would not alarm too many Christians, unaware that engaging in forms of meditation which induce altered states of consciousness is sufficient to create changes in one's belief system. The fact is that belief systems can be altered or challenged merely by doing tai chi and emptying one's mind.

Tom

Brenda Skyrme, a Christian counsellor in Lancashire UK who is experienced in dealing with people involved in Martial Arts, tells the story of Tom,[10] a young man who came to her seeking help. Tom's symptoms were:

- severe recurrent headaches
- an inability to remember what he had just read from the Bible.[11]

Tom had tried a number of sources to get help. He had approached members of his local church for advice and prayer without success. Finding no remedy, he sought medical help. His doctor placed him on *medication for tension and possible depression*, to no effect. His doctor then referred him to a specialist, who after testing him extensively, could find no cause for his problems.

In desperation and as a last resort, he sought help from Christian counsellors. After checking out his background, they put a question to him which no one had previously asked: *Have you ever been involved with anything occultist or any other faith system?*[12]

In his non-committal reply, Tom casually mentioned that he had been involved in tai chi chuan, the martial art form of tai chi. Brenda Skyrme related:

> His counsellors listened carefully knowing that the soft styles of Martial Arts in particular, could be the cause of headaches. Tom was then asked how he came to be involved. A friend had invited him to a class, he found the movements in tai chi interesting, and he enjoyed the peace of mind the exercises brought him. The emptying of all thoughts and anything that might distract him meant time away from daily problems.
>
> His counsellors explained the background of tai chi and the religious root, and how by making his mind a blank, he had allowed other forces to enter his unconscious. With him being a Christian, the confusion in some part was because his mind was trying to cope with two belief systems, and ungodly influences had entered his mind...
>
> After denouncing his involvement with the Martial Arts, he was able to be counselled and released from the ungodly influence that had caused his headaches and confusion.[13]

From Kung Fu to Christ

English evangelist Tony Anthony, in his autobiography, *Taming the Tiger*,[14] relates the remarkable story of his journey from Kung Fu World Champion to full-time evangelist for Christ, and makes it clear that it is impossible to be both a dedicated follower of chi and a devout follower of Christ.

At age four, Tony left his Chinese mother and Italian father in

England, to be placed under the care of his grandfather so that he might carry on the family tradition of Kung Fu. His grandfather, whom he addressed as Lowsi (master), was a Grand Master of the ancient art, and could trace his heredity back in a direct line to the famous Shaolin Temple, home of the Chinese martial arts.

Lowsi, who proved to be a demanding, even brutal taskmaster, first introduced him to tai chi, the foundation of Kung Fu. He recounts his early experiences: 'At first I could only watch as Lowsi performed his strange movements. He made me stand very still and breathe deeply, in through my nose and out through my mouth. It was mind numbingly tedious. As the weeks went by, and I began to pick up his language he explained his moves were Tai Chi, a discipline that is fundamental to the way of Kung Fu.'[15]

As well as *meditation in movement*, Lowsi taught him the art of chi kung, meditating in stillness, by getting him to gaze steadily at a flame for hours in a quiet corner of a temple:

> We spent hours in the temple, staring into the flame of a candle. I longed to close my eyes, but as they grew heavy, the thwack of bamboo hit my face. Lowsi beat me at any point he thought I was losing concentration. The purpose of these hours of meditation was to get in touch with the Chi. I was taught that all things are the products of cosmic negative and positive forces, the yin and the yang, which can be harmonised in the study of Chi. In the human body the Chi is best understood as the flow of energy. It is the Chi the disciples of the Tao believe governs muscular movement, the process of breathing, the regulation of the heartbeat and the functioning of the nervous system.

> 'When you can completely harmonise the Chi in both body and spirit, you will reach enlightenment [divinity] and inner peace. You will discover seemingly supernatural power within yourself', Lowsi taught me.

> 'Harnessing the Chi is essential in the art of Kung Fu', he continued, 'it allows for fluidity.'

Dipping his hand into a small vase of water he held it in the air until a small drop formed and lingered on the tip of his forefinger.

'A single drop of water. Alone, it is harmless, gentle and powerless. But what on earth can withstand the force of a Tsunami. Its raging waves have power to destroy earth and overcome all in its path. Learn to control the Chi, boy. Tap into its universal energy and you, too, will have power many times your natural strength.'

In the years ahead Lowsi's instruction in the Chi became clearer to me. I understood it to be the god within, the root of my power. Harnessing my body's energy through the chi, I could break bricks with my bare hands and perform much more amazing feats. It also gave me a heightened state of awareness, to the point where I could sense the movements of an opponent in the dark and withstand immense pain by distributing it throughout my body.[16]

By the time Tony was 17, he was so expert in the art of chi control and his ability in his martial skills, that he applied to become a Master of Kung Fu. His examination culminated in the notorious test of the tunnel, from which many never emerge alive.

Tony recounted one of the many death-defying hazards he encountered in this supreme test:

Next came the blade. It blocked my path and required me to walk along its razorsharp edge. In the torchlight I could see that the floor and walls around the obstacle were shimmering. 'Oil', I smiled. It covered the entirety of the rock. I was expected to walk the eight-metre blade to avoid the slippery surface. The cave walls were narrow at this point and there was no way around. I also sensed there was something more to this test. It would require the pinnacle of my concentration. I composed myself, harnessing the energy of the Chi into my feet so that I could feel no pain.

Keeping perfect balance, I stepped on the blade and began to walk. Suddenly, a wild and frenzied dog came tearing down the tunnel towards me. My master had drummed into me, 'Expect the unexpected.' Sure enough, in its madness it tried to lunge at me, but it was held back by a heavy chain. My control of the Chi ensured perfect calm. I continued to walk the blade.[17]

Now a Master of Kung Fu, Tony went on to become three times World Kung Fu Champion. From there he went on to become a security agent for some of the world's most powerful and influential people.

Later, as the pressures of life took their toll, he degenerated from being an enlightened Master to becoming a bloodthirsty and violent man, ending up in a hell-hole which was Cyprus's notorious Nicosia Central Prison. It was during his time there that he encountered a passionate Christian evangelist, Michael. During one of their sessions, Michael challenged Tony:

> 'All your life, you've had a God-shaped hole in your heart that you've been trying to fill,' Michael started. 'You've tried to fill it with Kung Fu, Buddhism; you've tried the glory of being a winner and being the best at your work; you've tried sex, drugs, anger, violence … None of these things have given you the satisfaction you crave. The one thing you have not tried is Jesus Christ … Tony, you've talked to me before about following the way of Kung Fu, but let me tell you, Jesus Christ said, "I am the way, the truth and the life. No one comes to the Father except through me." Kung Fu might claim to be a way; but he is the way. Just accept it, Tony.'[18]

Shortly after, Tony reached a point of sincere repentance. However, when the prison bully, Alcaponey, badly beat up his closest friend, Tony vowed to 'have' him in revenge. Accidentally they met each other in an isolated part of the jail. It was an immediate fight to the death. It was while they were in the very act of wrestling violently with each other, that Jesus spoke directly to Tony's heart: '*I am the way, the truth and the life*.'[19] At this, his desire to kill his enemy evaporated, and he heard himself uttering these words to Alcaponey; '*In the name of the Lord Jesus Christ, I command you to leave me alone*.'[20] Alcaponey left him immediately and did not return. Tony was gob-smacked: '*God had moved in a miraculous way, He had protected me and I hadn't even asked him to.*'[21]

After returning to his cell and still in a daze, he reflected on those words again:

> 'I am the way, the truth and the life' ... I feasted on the words and knew it had not been the Chi or martial arts that had saved me. It had been Jesus and my God-given faith that shielded me from clear and present danger. It was my first, most scariest, most powerful lesson in faith. I knew it was time to fully turn my back on the way of Kung Fu and put my trust firmly in the hands of God.[22]

Later, Tony was to look back at Kung Fu in light of that decisive event:

> From that incredible day when God demonstrated his power as I wrestled with Alcaponey, I have always discouraged people from any form of martial art. In the West it is mainly taught for fitness and self-defence, but it is rooted in spirituality that I believe is misleading and dangerous. Martial arts [including tai chi chuan] appeal to a person's fears, weaknesses and ego. Christ's way is to release a person into new life, freedom and security through, and in, him.[23]

Tony Anthony, ex Master of Kung Fu, one who once worshipped the god within and who had experienced a power from chi many times his natural strength, would have serious reservations with the claim that tai chi is not based on religious belief.

Psychic Powers

Tony Anthony's grandfather and mentor in martial tai chi once told him: 'When you can completely harmonise the Chi in both body and spirit you will reach enlightenment [divinisation] and inner peace. You will discover seemingly supernatural power within yourself.[24]

As Tony came to perform a range of amazing, *supernatural feats*, he became progressively convinced that he was divine. These powers he now possessed gave eloquent testimony to his divine nature – the *god within*. And such a path is open to anyone who seeks to become an adept of tai chi/chi kung. The supernatural powers most linked with tai chi are the powers of healing oneself and others, and amazing feats of strength commonly used in martial tai chi. But besides these, there is a wider range of psychic powers.

Supernatural Strength

Chi power, in its martial form, can manifest itself in many different ways. Tony Anthony, with his bare hands, was able to break bricks; in total darkness he was able to sense the movements of an opponent; when faced with physical dangers to his feet and hands he was *miraculously* able to nullify the dangers transferring extra chi to these parts of his body.

An interesting example of such chi power was presented in a British TV programme, *You Bet*, on 27th September, 1991. A martial arts student took up the challenge of breaking 100 roof tiles in one and a half minutes. The tiles were arranged in 20 piles of five each. Brenda Skyrme recounts:

> Before the challenge a chorus of shouts of 'kiai' went up from the assistants, answered by a similar shout from a competitor. This shouting continued with each shout becoming greater in volume and strength. Suddenly the shouting stopped. The chi power had been built up and the competition started. The sequence of action was fast and violent. All of the tiles were broken within the required time of one and half minutes.

> It so happened that an interested engineer decided to replay the action of this event very slowly so as to observe the competitor's action in breaking the tiles. To the engineer's total amazement, he discovered that in fact the tiles were never touched; the force of

the chi power broke the tiles without ever coming into contact
with the competitor's hand. That was the force and power of chi.[25]

'Miraculous' Healing through Chi

Some grandmasters make many claims about the healing powers of
tai chi. The sceptics may attribute such healing to the simple fact of
regular exercise of every part of the body rather than to the power
of a spiritual force called chi. But to highlight the supernatural nature
of the healing power of tai chi, I have selected a few examples of
dramatic healings which defy rational explanation.

Wolfe Lowenthal narrates how his distinguished tai chi teacher,
Professor Cheng, healed himself of a seemingly fatal disease through
tai chi. In his twenties, Professor Cheng developed tuberculosis.
Lowenthal relates:

> His doctors predicted that he had six months to live; Professor
> Cheng took up the art of Tai Chi Chuan [martial tai chi] in a last
> ditch effort to save his life. Soon he stopped coughing blood, his
> fever left and the tuberculosis was cured. He was still prone to ill
> health but would later consider that a blessing, because whenever
> he was tempted to give up the arduous study of Tai Chi Chuan, he
> would get sick and only the resumption of his Tai Chi would cure
> him. So he persevered.[26`]

Practising tai chi for the rest of his life, he remained free of the
dreaded tuberculosis.

The Cobra Strikes Again!

In tai chi, great emphasis is placed on the importance of moving chi
quickly to different parts of the body according to need. A particular
type of movement of chi closely parallels the movement of prana as
expressed in the arousing of the kundalini.

Lowenthal relates what appears to be a description of kundalini arousal in the context of tai chi, from a lecture by his hero, Professor Cheng:

> Chinese medicine puts great emphasis on the development of the chi. The chi circulates like blood, and the tan tien is the seat of chi. The tan tien is located 3.25cm below the navel, 0.75cm from the front of the body, 1.75cm from the back.
>
> The chi accumulates from the tan tien by means of blood vessels, membranes, the space between membranes and the tendons. Circulating through the body, the chi pulls the blood, like a horse pulls a chariot.[27]

Cheng then describes a process which occurs in the context of tai chi:

> A man begins this process with seminal fluid created in the uro-genital system. This fluid goes to the tan tien where it joins with the chi of the blood, directed into the tan tien by the will. Then you breathe in the chi of heaven and direct it to the tan tien. The seminal chi, called ching chi, gathers in the tan tien with the chi of the blood and the chi of the heavens. Staying there long enough, they will come to generate a kind of steam, something like electricity. This steam flows out of the tan tien, through the sacrum and into the spine and bones, where it condenses into a paper thin tissue. This type of marrow gradually fills the bones, causing them to become hard like steel. Then it flows up the spine to the brain and finally returns to the tan tien.
>
> You should pay special attention to the Yellow Emperor's words, 'The Sage swallows the chi of heaven to achieve spiritual enlightenment'. This is also the process whereby a sage can sit alone in his room and **come to know everything**[28] (emphasis added).

Professor Cheng's description of chi kundalini has a number of features in common with yogic kundalini. Both take their origin from sexual energy. The production of this energy is accompanied by a sensation of heat. In both there is an energy transfer from the base of the spine to the crown of the head. Both forms result in *spiritual enlightenment*, the attainment of divinity, which is accompanied by, indeed proved by, a range of psychic powers. Cheng expresses this range succinctly in his statement: *a sage can sit alone in his room and come to know everything.*

The Chinese shamanic tradition is captured in the use of the word sage. It included contact with the spirit world, the ability to know the past and predict the future, astral projection, the interpretation of *spirit-dreams*, and healing. Here we have a parallel with the *siddhis* of yoga.

7

Taoist Philosophy

Tai chi is based solely on a philosophy. But that philosophy, Taoism, is in reality a system of religious beliefs. It answers such perennial religious questions as:

- Who made the world?
- Is there a supreme being?
- What is the purpose of life?
- What happens after death?
- How does one surrender to the supreme being?
- How can one become a healer?
- How can one predict the future?
- What is the morally good life?

Taoist philosophy gives us direct answers, the acceptance of which requires religious faith.

Tai chi and chi kung, in fact, are powerful ways of nurturing the faith which stems from Taoist philosophy. An adept of these arts develops a strong, personal faith in chi, which lacks the usual trappings of a religion, such as a temple, a priestly hierarchy, worship in common and the like. The temple now becomes a local hall, ironically often a Christian church hall or retreat centre; masters and their staff become the religious priests and teachers; the class going through the routine of graceful movements becomes the communal worship and means of surrender to the Supreme Ultimate of Chi. And one's private devotion is nurtured in the intimacy of the lounge room as one gazes at the white-robed figures on video, seeking to imitate their graceful movements and inner focus. Some New Age followers may not be too keen on the discipline required to perfect such movements, but they are captivated by a philosophy which promises to one day give them entrance to the hall of the gods. And this philosophy is captured in two classic works.

The I Ching (Book of Changes)

Taoist philosophy has its roots in the misty origins of Chinese shamanism. These shamans were spiritual leaders who specialised in a 'trance-dance' which enabled them 'to communicate with the dead, demons and nature spirits.'[1] From such sources they received revelations which over thousands of years formed collectively a fund of spiritual wisdom and was eventually committed to writing as the I Ching about 1000 B.C. It is regarded as the first great classic of Taoism.

The book gives us a systematic account of the theory of yin-yang in terms of all the phenomena occurring in both the cosmos and the human person – past, present and future. Its primary use has been as a medium for predicting the future for which its adherents claim great success. A key to understanding the I Ching is 'The Eight Diagrams'.

Figure 2. The Eight Diagrams.

In the trigrams in the sketch below, an unbroken line = yang, two broken lines = yin, and in this way the eight trigrams:

- collectively represent the whole of reality
- collectively indicate the tendencies of things in movement.

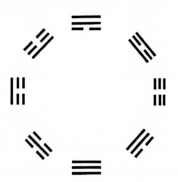

Tai chi has been strongly influenced by these eight diagrams. Each of the eight basic moves in tai chi corresponds to one of the eight diagrams.

It is worthy of note that the ecstatic state in which the shamans received their revelations for the I Ching was known as 'illumined spirit'. It is this same state which is the core goal of tai chi and chi kung.

The Tao Te Ching (pron. dow day ching)

As a book of Taoist philosophy, the I Ching was superseded some 700 years later by a book which is regarded as the 'bible' of Taoism, the Tao Te Ching. It is attributed to Lao Tsu, a shamanic sage who lived during the sixth century BC. However, not published till ~ 300 B.C., the work is now considered to be the work of a group of disciple-scholars of Lao Tsu.

That this text should be considered a source of revelation is not surprising. Firstly, it took as its starting point the I Ching. Secondly, it was the product of 'a society that had a strong shamanic culture' which greatly influenced Lao Tsu and his disciples. Reverential mention is made to sages in the pages of the text, and these sages were in fact shamans.

More than any other book, it was the Tao Te Ching which shaped the development of tai chi particularly through its system of religious beliefs summarised in its description of creation.

Figure 3. Taoist Theory of Creation

Taoists believe that the stillness of nothingness (wu chi) gave rise to the motion (yang) and the stillness (yin) of Tai Chi, which gave rise to the whole of creation (Cosmic Chi). In the Tai Chi fish symbol, there always exists an element of yin in yang and vice versa. And note the descent of chi into the universe.

The Tao and Wu Chi are different names for the same reality. Wu Chi, sometimes referred to as 'The Great Infinite Void', is not so much a state of nothingness but rather one of infinite potential which

CREATION

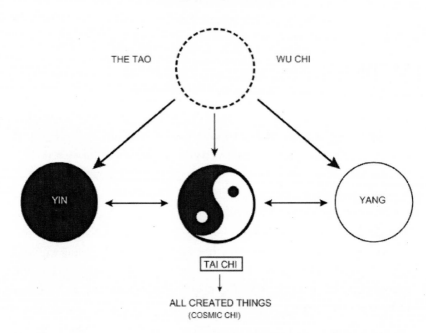

is the ultimate source of all creation. Our universe began when Wu Chi gave rise to motion (yang) alternating with stillness (yin). Perfect harmony between these two complementary forces produced the state of Tai Chi (a philosophical concept spelt in this text with capital letters to distinguish it from the exercise 'tai chi' spelt with lower case). Wu Chi and Tai Chi are considered to be one and the same reality under different forms, though the void of Wu Chi is regarded as the higher state to which one aspires when voiding one's mind in performing tai chi and chi kung.

The Attributes of Wu Chi

Wu Chi is presented as an impersonal, benevolent energy which gives rise to the equally impersonal forces of yin and yang which comprise chi, aptly referred to in *Star Wars* as 'The Force'.

Wu Chi is the eternal supreme creator of the universe:

> *All things arise from the Tao.*[2]
> *It is the forefather of the gods (and spirits).*[3]

In order to follow the way of the Tao it is essential to have a religious faith which accepts the Tao as the supreme deity:

> *The greatest virtue is to follow Tao and Tao alone.*
> *Oh it is dim and dark and yet within is essence.*
> *This essence is very real and therein lies faith.*[4]

In this faith the committed Taoist will leave behind all other gods including Jesus Christ, as did Tony Anthony during his Kung Fu phase, in order to follow the Tao alone. And in doing so with perseverance and helped by tai chi, one will 'attain the divine'.

Tai Chi

This philosophical concept is comprised of yin and yang. Some of the attributes of yin and yang are shown in the table below:

Yin	Yang
Destructive	Constructive
Passive	Active
Cold	Hot
Soft	Hard
Dark	Light
Low	High
Moon	Sun
Stillness	Movement
Feminine	Masculine
Water	Fire
Earth	Sky

Since Taoism seeks to explain all reality in terms of yin and yang, we could extend the table above to include all moral behaviour and classify virtues and vices into yin and yang. One complementary couple would be love (yang) and hate (yin). In Taoism, love and hate cannot be categorised as good and evil respectively since there is always a small amount of hate in love and vice versa. Moreover, love and hate in any given person are constantly interacting and changing.

What this means in reality is that in Taoism there are no moral absolutes, all is relative, and the terms 'good' and 'evil' as used in the Christian tradition have no place in this philosophy. As the Taoist adepts reach a state of enlightenment, they create their own morality which it is believed will be the way of Nature, whatever that may mean.

Cosmic Chi

Tai Chi purportedly gave rise to all creatures in the universe. In this act, chi creates by extending itself in the same way that Brahman extends itself through prana. So everything in nature – trees, whales, the stars, humans – are all in essence chi. As Professor Cheng would say, 'The chi that flows in our bodies is the same chi that moves the stars in the heavens.'[5] This belief that the supreme god chi is everything and everything is chi is know as **pantheism**. And since all creatures share the same essence chi, it follows that there is an extraordinary oneness in the the cosmos – one is all and all is one. This belief of **monism** excludes all dualities such as that between the ego and the spirit, between the spiritual and material, and between good and evil.

Personal Chi

Within this belief system, humans are a unique manifestation of chi and are born in a state of original innocence called the *state of the uncarved block*.[6] Just as an uncarved block has limitless potential in the hands of a gifted craftsperson, echoing the infinite potential of Wu Chi, so do humans at the time of birth with their original supply of personal Wu Chi. As life progresses, this original innocence quickly becomes tainted, and the initial supply of personal chi suffers a corresponding reduction. In Taoist thought, the whole purpose of life is to recapture original innocence by cultivating and storing ever-new supplies of chi. The meditation in motion of tai chi and the meditation in stillness of chi kung are considered excellent means of converting cosmic chi into personal chi.

Chi is sometimes described as the *animating force* in the universe. It gives all things existence. In terms of humans, it is often referred to as the *life force* or soul. It is well to remember that **this life force is in fact divine**. Hence, in humans, the chi is the god within, the divine spark. The purpose of life is to fan this spark into a blazing furnace.

Ardent disciples of the Tao who reach this point, become one with the Tao. During this life, their reward is good health and a long life. At death, they become an *immortal*, one with the Tao, and are revered by Taoists as sages.

Death to the Ego

We have seen earlier how the monistic philosophy underpinning yoga results in the dissolution of the 'illusory' ego. A similar monistic strand, implicit in early Taoism, became much more explicit through the influence of Buddhism. The philosopher Jacob Needleman, in his insightful commentary on the Tao Te Ching, expresses the view that the ego is 'an ephemeral construction'[7] and through the type of meditation practised in tai chi and chi kung will eventually be annihilated: *At every state of the practice [of meditation] the truth one needs to experience is 'hidden' and 'dark' and bears the marks of 'death'. This is the death of all that has been built up by the automatism of the mind and ego.*[8]

8

To Chi or not to Chi?

Currently in Australia, many Christians including ministers, priests and religious practise tai chi. It is offered at Christian retreat centres, in church halls, on staff spirituality days in Catholic schools. So is tai chi compatible with Christianity? My answer is a definite No.

I believe that Christians who become involved in tai chi are placing themselves in serious spiritual danger. Orthodox Christians would perceive the philosophy which undergirds tai chi as the worship of a false god which results in the tai chi adept developing occult powers in the pursuit of becoming divine. Even if one seeks to distance oneself from the chi philosophy, the techniques involved in this meditation in movement are such as to significantly alter the practitioner's state of consciousness. The empty mind and passive will involved in this state expose the practitioner to demonic influence, and in the advanced state of 'enlightenment', even to possession.

Blowing the Mind

The way of becoming perfectly united to the void of Wu Chi is to become a void oneself. The way this void is reached is through simple mind-altering techniques. The first deep-relaxation technique is slow, rhythmic breathing which permeates all the practitioner's movements. This lessens the chatter of the mind.

A second more powerful relaxant is a form of meditation peculiar to tai chi. It involves meditation **in** movement and meditation **on** movement. The mind visualises each movement as it is being performed to capture the feel and nature of it. Since the mind is totally focused on the bodily expression of some aspect of nature, the chatter of the mind becomes greatly reduced through the sequence of movements. Combined with the slow, rhythmical movement of the 'dance', this induces in the practitioner a form of trance. Cohen notes the similarity of this 'dance-trance' to that of the ancient Chinese shamanic dances, the purpose of which was to make contact with the spirit world: 'Many of today's [tai chi] exercises are sets of linked postures, each flowing into the next, as in a beautiful slow motion dance. Inspired by ancient ritual dances [they are] designed to alter consciousness.'[1]

It is important to note that this trance can be reached by following these techniques without believing in the religious system which is Taoist philosophy.

Chi Cheats Christ

Commitment to tai chi inevitably undermines one's faith in Christ because the system of religious beliefs underpinning tai chi is at loggerheads with Christian beliefs.

A serious warning of the dangers of becoming involved in martial arts based on the power of chi, comes from Bill Rudge, the founder of the Christian Martial Arts Association (USA). After many years teaching martial arts, Bill decided to abandon all involvement and made his reasons public. One reason particularly applied to tai chi:

> His fourth reason involves the Martial Arts connection between Eastern mysticism [Taoist philosophy] and the occult. He observes that many people who begin innocently, using the martial arts merely for self defence, physical discipline, health benefits, or sports competition, eventually become involved in occult practice and philosophy.[2]

Another reason Rudge gave for abandoning martial arts was the pride to which it gave rise:

> Many claim humility, but I believe it is a false, deceptive humility. I began to think I was god and almost invincible. I became haughty and egotistical and had an air of superiority when dealing with people. And I saw the same attitude in almost every student and instructor (even Christians). Many impressionable students (even advanced practitioners) idolised and practically worshipped their senseis [teachers] and masters.[3]

The Nature of Chi

Some Christians maintain that chi is just another name for the God of Christianity. And indeed, chi and the Holy Trinity have certain characteristics in common – they are both infinite, eternal, creators of all things. However, there are fundamental differences. Chi is an impersonal power, whereas the God of Christians is essentially personal. The Trinity is three Persons in intimate, loving communion with each other. This God of infinite love has reached out in love to create humans. And when our first parents sinned, God the Father sent his Son to redeem us by taking human flesh and becoming one with us. Such passionate love is quite different to the detached benevolence of *the Force*, or the emptiness of *the Void*.

Another significant difference between the Christian God and chi is the nature of their respective creations. Creation by chi is both pantheistic and monistic. The Christian God, while being in all creatures to sustain them in existence, is quite separate in identity to them all. To orthodox Christians, Taoism is simply the worship of a false god which frequently ends up as the worship of nature. It is not without significance that tai chi devotees turn to face the rising sun, supposedly the richest expression of chi in our immediate world.

The Australian Idol

If at one time Taoism was a form of Chinese idolatry, it is no longer peculiar to that race. Over recent years it has spread rapidly throughout the Western world, and has made its presence felt strongly in Australia. Idolatry is not new to the People of God. It has been a continuing temptation through the ages. Today, the attraction to idol worship through tai chi is so subtle that it is duping many Christians, even their leaders.

In St Paul's day, idolatry took an obvious form in the worship of statues of gods in the temples. Today, while it comes disguised as a source of good health and a stress-free life, the stern warning which Paul gave his flock remains relevant: 'Does this mean that food sacrificed to idols has a real value, or that the idol itself is real? Not at all. It simply means that the sacrifices that they offer, they sacrifice to demons who are not God. I have no desire to see you in communion with demons. You cannot drink the cup of the Lord and the cup of demons.'[4]

The tai chi-er who makes a total surrender of mind and heart to the cosmic chi is performing a personal act of worship to a non-existent idol which masks demonic powers, and in doing so, runs the serious danger of being *in communion with demons*. Should such a person be approaching the altar of the Lord?

Original Innocence v Original Sin

While the shamanic revelation of Taoism presents the new-born as being in an idyllic state, Christian revelation presents us with a markedly different picture of the state of the newborn, a picture which has its origins in the dawn of the human race and is outlined in the figurative language of the book of Genesis which nevertheless *affirms a primeval event, a deed that took place at the beginning of the history of man.*[5]

This account narrates how our first parents, Adam and Eve, were created in a state of holiness, sharing the divine life of God, and living in a state of perfect harmony with God, with themselves, with each other and with creation. While in this state of original innocence, we are told, they deliberately succumbed to a sin of disobedience which deprived them of God's life and destroyed the harmony of humans with God, with themselves, with each other and with the created cosmos. Sadly, the effects of this sin have been transmitted to all the descendants of Adam and Eve through the collective bond of human nature: Adam and Eve transmitted to their descendants human nature flawed by their own first sin – a deprivation called 'original sin'.[6] *As a result of original sin, human nature*, according to the *Catholic Catechism*, *is weakened in its powers; subject to ignorance, suffering and the domination of death; and inclined to sin.*[7]

Paul, speaking collectively of the human race, speaks of the effects of original sin: 'I do not understand my own behaviour, I do not act as I mean to, but I do things I hate.'[8] Paul is also keenly aware that the solution to his dilemma is close at hand. 'Who will rescue me from this body doomed to death? God – thanks be to him – through Jesus Christ our Lord.'[9]

The Taoist concept of enlightenment, therefore, and the Christian concept of salvation are diametrically opposed. Taoism claims to turn people into gods; Christianity offers transformation of humans into images of Christ, while they still remain creatures. It can be clearly seen that tai chi, one means of achieving Taoist salvation, is not only seriously at odds with the Christian way, but is an alternative system of salvation which does away with the need for Christ.

Suspect Supernatural Powers

Through the combination of mind altering techniques and the worshipful surrender to the false god of chi, tai chi adepts have shown themselves capable of developing a variety of super-human powers which defy rational explanation. These include feats of extraordinary physical, aggressive strength; seemingly miraculous healings, predicting the future, reading minds, astral projection, communing with the spirit world as exemplified by exponents of chi kundalini.

Altered states of consciousness exposing one to demonic influence combined with idol worship inducing communion with demons, combine powerfully in tai chi to produce such supernatural powers. To the superficial observer, such powers may appear identical to the Christian charismatic gifts of the Holy Spirit. And indeed, there is a remarkable parallel, for Satan is able to counterfeit all of the Christian charismatic gifts. If an individual is able to exercise a package of such 'gifts', and some of them are clearly contrary to biblical teaching, such, for example as divination using the I Ching or channelling, then it is highly likely that the other 'gifts' in the package are occultic. Suffice to say that if such extraordinary gifts are exercised by someone claiming either to be a god or on the path to divinity, then such gifts come not from the Spirit of God but from Satan. 'There appears to be little difference between the mystical energy (chi) in the martial arts (e.g., tai chi chuan) and the psychic energy used by the occultist, whether shaman, witch doctor, medium, spiritistic channeller, or psychic healer.'[10]

Ego-Destruct

Taoist forms of meditation such as the *meditation in movement* of tai chi and the *meditation in stillness* of chi kung, have developed with the express intention of reducing the human person to a non-ego state. In popular language, the ego includes the intellect, the will and the emotions, each of which makes a special contribution to the formation of a unique personality. Taoist meditation produces a gradual dissolution of these three faculties by habitually emptying the mind to the point where its critical faculties are suspended in a 'void'. The suspension of the critical faculties produces a paralysis of the will which leaves it exposed to whatever forces are 'out there'. In such an extreme passive state, the emotions too become increasingly suppressed.

As witnessed repeatedly with yoga, when such passive states become extreme, the so-called state of higher consciousness produced leaves the adept exposed to demonic influence, an exposure which is heightened when the process is accompanied by surrender to a demonic spirit(s) hiding behind the mask of a false god, chi.

When carried to the point of "enlightenment", the old personality is completely blown away and a totally new personality shaped by demonic powers emerges.

Ego-Construct

Christianity, far from dismissing the ego as an illusory appendage to the spirit or a blockage to spiritual development, embraces it as an integral part of the human person and, as such, an instrument of salvation and sanctification.

To appreciate the part the ego plays in human development from the Christian perspective, we need to reflect on the origin of the human race described in Genesis:

> God created man in the image of himself, in the image of God he created him, male and female he created them. God blessed them, saying to them, 'Be fruitful, multiply, fill the earth and subdue it. Be masters of the fish of the sea, the birds of heaven and all the living creatures that move on the earth' ... God saw all that he had made, and indeed it was very good.[11]

This creation account is charged with implication concerning the place of the ego in human personality. Humans are created in 'the image of God' with the capacity to:

- know and self-reflect
- exercise free will
- experience a range of emotions.

Collectively, these faculties constitute the human ego. And since God's word tells us that all of God's creation, including the human person, is *very good*, it follows that these three constituents of the ego are also *very good*. Even after original sin, the human ego, though weakened and disordered, is still essentially good. And it can be progressively purified and strengthened by the redeeming power of Christ through justification and sanctification.

Indeed, the first commandment of Christianity binds Christians to use their ego as an instrument for loving God. When Jesus was questioned by the Pharisees as to *what was the greatest commandment of the Law*, (Mt 22:36) he responded. *You must love the Lord your God with all your heart ... .*[12]

Now the word *heart* in this context embraces the will, the intellect and the emotions – all important instruments for loving God.

A Personal God

People tend to become like the god they worship. In worshipping a personal God, Christians do so in a personal way. Christians seek to love their God with all their heart, and in New Testament usage, the heart comes close to meaning 'the person' as C Ryder Smith contends: 'It (the heart) does not altogether lose its physical reference for it is made of 'flesh' (2 Cor 3:3), but it is the seat of the will (e.g., Mk 3:5), of the intellect (e.g., Mk 2:6-8), and of feeling (e.g., Lk 24:32). This means that 'heart' comes the nearest of the New Testament terms to mean 'person'.[13]

True Christians, then, bring their whole person to the service and worship of God. In so doing, they form themselves in the likeness of the personal God they worship. Those who take tai chi and chi kung seriously, in aiming to nullify their ego, shape themselves after the impersonal god they worship – *The Force*.

Tai minus Chi and ASC.

Some Christians involved in tai chi claim that they neither accept the philosophy of chi nor perform any mind-altering techniques. Any tai chi master would deplore such a hollowed-out version of the art. In fact, such a person is not performing tai chi but rather a graceful form of callisthenics. If one is performing this neutered version in private and not watching a tai chi video, there seems to me no spiritual danger. If, however, one is performing in this way as a member of a tai chi class, then one can be influenced unconsciously by the occult power emanating from the teacher or others in the class.

I am aware of tai chi being taught in physical education programmes in some Christian schools. The students may be taught the various movements but not the accompanying philosophy. However, if such introductory classes involve retarded breathing and meditation on the movements, there are real spiritual dangers. Even if participation is confined strictly to the movements, there is a danger that students will carry a wrong message into later life: 'If tai chi was part of the curriculum in a Christian school, it must be O.K!' And with this dangerous message in their minds, alumni may later engage in an activity which they were "told" by their teachers was innocent.

Part C

REIKI

9

A Crypto-Religion

About 20 years ago, I received a phone call from a woman in Sydney who had just completed a course in Christian prayer with me. She told me that she had been invited to a weekend seminar on Reiki (ray key) which, she explained, was a form of healing through the laying on of hands. Never having heard of Reiki, I asked questions. She said that after completing the seminar she would automatically receive the power to heal. My spiritual antennas went up. A short time later I came across a large poster in a health shop window, advertising a Reiki seminar and giving an all-too-brief account of what would occur at the seminar, but very clear about the final result:

Do this seminar and become a healer! Having completed this seminar, it claimed, you could later progress to do an advanced course which would automatically give you the ability to heal at a distance.

Turn the clock forward 15 years and Reiki was no longer a rarity in Australia. It was widespread and big business. The internet, New Age magazines and holistic health journals were full of ads. Hundreds of Reiki practitioners are found in all major cities.

Across the world there are more than 200,000 Reiki Masters in Western countries and thousands of different schools with a wide diversity of approaches.

One of Reiki's leading proponents, Frank Petter, claims that 'Reiki has become the most frequently applied individual healing technique throughout the world.'[1] He forecasts: 'Reiki has spread all over the globe within a period of 20 years, and it will spread into the hearts of many more of our fellow human beings in the new millennium.'[2]

The Ancient Healing Art

The name *reiki* is composed of two Japanese words *rei* and *ki*. *Rei* means universal and *ki* means *chi*. So Reiki is literally *universal divine energy*. Most Reiki people regard Reiki as The Source, a supreme god in much the same way as Taoists regard Wu Chi, as Hindus regard Brahman (prana), as Christians regard Christ. And indeed it is interesting to note that the name of the supreme god of Shingon Buddhism, the religion of Mikao Usui, the founder of modern Reiki, is *Universal Divine Energy*!

Klaudia Hochhuth, a Reiki Master operating out of Ballarat in Victoria, provides us with a handy definition of Reiki:

'Reiki is an ancient art of natural healing rediscovered in Japan over 100 years ago. What is described as Reiki – the Usui System of Natural Healing – can be defined as follows:

- It is a gentle, but powerful 'hands-on' technique, which brings wholeness to both recipient and giver.
- It restores the natural balance in the body.
- It provides deep relaxation, thus evoking a sense of peace and well-being.
- It works on the emotions, mind and spirit as well as the physical body.
- It complements – but does not substitute for – the healing properties of orthodox medical treatment, natural therapies, and massage.
- It is not intrusive, since the Reiki energy will pass through clothing, bandages, braces, plaster casts, etc., so that no disrobing is necessary.
- It has no connection with any religion, cult, dogma, or special belief system and does not involve hypnosis or massage.
- The technique can be used not only on people, but also on animals and plants.
- To benefit from Reiki you only need to be open and willing to receive the energy. Everyone can learn it.'[3]

This prompts a number of questions:

- What is the ultimate source of this "natural" healing?
- How similar is the "laying on of hands" in Reiki to the "laying on of hands" in Christian healing?
- Does "being open" mean surrendering to any spiritual power 'out there'?

For many, their first introduction to Reiki is a **full-body treatment** to promote general health – physical, mental, emotional and spiritual.

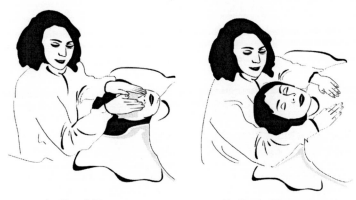

A. Head Treatment   B. Body Treatment

Dressed in normal clothing, the recipient lies face upward on a massage table. The Reiki practitioner stands behind the head of the recipient and places both hands on the recipient's forehead and eyes. After transmitting Reiki there for a few minutes, the practitioner places his/her hands at each side of the head near the temples with fingers covering each ear. Once again, Reiki is transmitted for a few minutes. After this, both hands are placed under the recipient's head, cradling it while Reiki is transmitted. Next, the practitioner places the fingers of both hands lightly on the throat, completing the head treatment.

The practitioner then moves to the recipient's side, placing his/her hands over the heart, then the lower rib cage, the navel and finally the groin. The recipient then turns over to face downwards. The practitioner gives the Reiki treatment with both hands successively to the shoulders, the middle back, the kidneys and pelvis. Some practitioners also treat the knees and feet.

Depending on the practitioner, such a basic treatment may take anywhere between an hour and 90 minutes. If the practitioner senses that there is an energy imbalance in some part of the body, then Reiki may be transmitted to that area for some time.

Such a session is frequently accompanied by:

- quiet soft music
- the burning of incense
- subdued lighting.

If the practitioner considers it advisable, the practitioner's hands, instead of touching the recipient's body, may be held a few centimetres above the skin. The effect is the same.

Recipients respond to Reiki healing in various ways. Some experience:

- a strong surge of energy through the body
- a warm tingling throughout the body or in certain parts
- a feeling of relaxation
- falling sound asleep
- perspiring heavily
- an emotional release accompanied by crying
- the lessening of pain in a hurting part of the body
- feeling very little at all.

Self-Healing

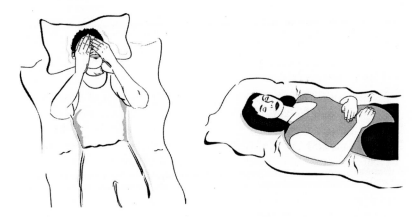

A. Self Treatment: Head   B. Self Treatment: Body

Once people have been initiated into the first level of Reiki, they are strongly encouraged to give themselves Reiki for 15 to 30 minutes daily for the purpose of:

- maintaining and increasing good health[4]
- growing in self-love[5]
- improving one's emotional life[6]
- relaxing more deeply[7]
- engaging more easily in forms of meditation which eliminate mental chatter and
- feelings and create an experience of harmony and joy[8]
- nurturing one's own spiritual life by making contact with the Higher Self (the divine Self).[9]

Despite the fact that Reiki universally presents itself as a spirituality acceptable to a secular society, the health profession and all religions, I believe it is a de-institutionalised religious system because:

- Usui Reiki takes its origin from a blend of Taoist and Buddhist religious beliefs.

- Usui Reiki takes its origin from a supernatural revelation underpinned by Buddhism.

- The Reiki movement has its own dogmas and morality.

- Reiki offers a form of supernatural healing.

- The form of religion presented by Reiki is both un-biblical and anti-Christian.

- The practice of Reiki generally leads to the acquiring of certain supernatural powers which are demonic in origin. **Because its practitioners cover or cloud the true nature of this system, and because it does not have the usual trappings of a formalised religion, I refer to Reiki as a crypto-religion which nestles comfortably into New Age**.

Empowered by the divine

The origin of Reiki as practised in the traditional Usui System in the West lies in the recent past. This form of supernatural healing was discovered just over a century ago by a 34-year-old Japanese man, Mikao Usui. Usui's journey to Reiki was fascinating, beginning some eleven years before he "discovered" Reiki, or before Reiki "discovered" him in 1899.

In his youth, Usui, like many young Japanese, had traded his Buddhist faith for the great god of scientific knowledge as he pursued a career of Western medicine. He was already a qualified medical doctor when he had the first experience which launched him on a new life-path. Without warning, he was suddenly smitten by deadly cholera. The treatment he was given was current at the time in Japan – small balls of opium placed beneath the tongue.

This, however, did little to improve his condition. His health degenerated rapidly to the point where his doctor announced that he would not survive the night. Usui was written off as dead and lapsed into a coma, partly induced by the delirium of his cholera and partly by the effects of his opiate. Sometime later he felt that he was "awakening" from this coma. In fact he was experiencing a vision of the Buddhist heaven where he saw countless Buddhas in glory. As far as Usui was concerned his most significant encounter was with Medicine King Buddha, the Buddha most concerned with healing in all its forms. Usui gives us an account of their meeting:

> At that time Medicine King Buddha spoke to me and said I was a physician as he was, and that it would be my job, my mission, when I had recovered from my illness, to work to make a synthesis of both teachings [the Western and the Buddhist]. At that time he expressed to me the age old teaching that the life energy, the Hari [the chi collected in the tan tien], is not separate from the body and that all physical suffering first emanates from the Hari and is due to karmic obscuration and past actions, which lead to suffering. The surgeon's knife or the physician's pill can only temporarily relieve this suffering. For the individual to be truly healed, he must be healed of ignorance, hatred and greed. He must live a moral life, carefully walking the Middle Path and seeking enlightenment for his own self and others; that is the only true healing, that the Dharma [the teaching and practices of Buddhism] is the **only** balm and medicine for the suffering of all living beings[10] (emphasis added).

Certain beliefs expressed by Medicine King Buddha remain current in Western Usui Reiki today:

- karma and reincarnation
- illness commences in the tan tien and only later manifests in the body
- among Reiki leaders, the main object of Reiki is the pursuit of enlightenment or becoming divine; healings are a by-product of this.

Having completed his teaching on healing, Medicine King Buddha aimed a 'healing laser' of blue light from his heart to Usui's body, upon which Usui lapsed into unconsciousness. To the great astonishment of his doctor, Usui woke up next morning completely healed of his cholera.[11]

After this vision and 'miraculous healing', Usui had a religious conversion to Shingon Buddhism. The whole purpose of his life now became to seek enlightenment through Buddhist teaching and the practice of Buddhist healing. In this pursuit, he joined a spiritualist society called Rei Jyutsu Ka which practice enabled him to make contact with the spirits of the dead and presumably with his Buddhist deities.

In his research into Buddhist healing Usui discovered a secret method of healing which he believed originated with the historical Gautama Buddha. After experimenting with this method without success, he determined to make a pilgrimage to Mt Kurama, a Buddhist sacred site in which there was a Buddhist temple and a centre of the spiritualist society of which Usui was a member.

Usui's visit to Mt. Kurama would prove to be his second pivotal experience. During his 21 day retreat, Usui had a profound experience in which he perceived certain images and felt empowered to use them in the cause of healing. He related: 'These spheres manifested before me like bubbles rising on water and then I became aware of their importance and the methodology with which to employ them...[they] sank into me and bestowed on me the power to impart this healing modality to everyone.'[12]

Initially, the ability to impart this healing power rested with Usui alone. Later, others were to be able to impart it, but only as a result of an empowerment by Usui. This marked the beginning of a spiritual lineage with Usui as the patriarch, a lineage that has continued from Master to Master to our own day. According to Reiki's practitioners, if the lineage is broken, the power of Reiki is not handed on.

Empowered on the mountain-top, Usui descended to the market-place, seemingly possessed of a strong gift of healing. Following the instructions of his vision years earlier, he began to initiate his Buddhist disciples into this same power. Over 20 years the demand for his Reiki healers steadily grew and eventually became so great that he developed a form for non-Buddhists. It was this so-called non-religious form, considerably modified, which was eventually transported to the West after his death. It contains the four symbols revealed to Usui.

The Sacred Symbols

These symbols are used in the three levels of Reiki – Levels 1 and 2 and Master's. Reiki people believe that the correct usage and the correct drawing of the symbols is essential for the transmission of the Reiki power. Because these symbols are the means of making contact with the source of Reiki, the ultimate divinity, great reverence is devoted to drawing the symbols to activate them. Ellyard stresses: 'Each time we sign a Reiki symbol we are signing the name of the sacred. In doing so we honour the divinity of the universal energy and we honour ourselves.'[13]

Because of the sacred nature of these symbols, until recently they were kept a closely guarded secret in the Reiki culture. However the last decade has seen a growing tendency to publish them.

The psychic insertion of the four classic Usui symbols is the key to Reiki power and there is a commonly accepted version of each of the symbols in the Reiki culture. The four symbols are written as Japanese characters. I have substituted my own English shorthand for each of the symbols:

The Power Symbol (P)

This symbol brings the power of Reiki to a particular place and is often used in conjunction with the other three symbols to boost their effect.

The Mental Emotional Symbol (E)

This symbol clears any mental, emotional and addictive blockages, and thus improves one's relationships with people.

The Long Distance Symbol

This symbol enables one to transmit Reiki to any person, place or event in any part of the world; to transmit Reiki to past/future events in one's current life or in one's supposed previous lives and to make contact with 'angelic' spirit guides, spirits of the dead or deities. In this respect, I refer to this as the spiritualistic symbol.

The Master Symbol

The use of this symbol makes it patently clear that Reiki involves the worship of a supreme deity. It is an invocation of the universal life energy which, according to Petter, 'is an absolute truth and transcends the differences between all religions'.[14]

Reiki Initiations

While the public are becoming increasingly aware of Reiki, few outside the culture know what is involved in the process of getting 'the power'. Most Masters see the initiation experience as a sacred ritual giving the initiate 'a more immediate experience of the divine'.[15] They maintain that the only way to appreciate Reiki initiation is to be initiated and that the rite cannot be comprehended by outsiders. Unlike yoga and tai chi, very little is explained about how to tap in. Only a small number of Masters in more recent times have been prepared to reveal any of the secrets behind the *power*.

Usui Reiki Western System, the so-called non-religious kind, has three levels:

> Level 1 involves four initiations and empowers one to channel Reiki to oneself and others by placing the hands on different parts of the body. This makes one a Reiki Practitioner.
>
> Level 2 involves one initiation which empowers one to use three symbols, P, E and D, enabling one to give distance Reiki.
>
> Level 3 involves one initiation which empowers one to initiate

others into Reiki at all three levels, and empowers one to use the M symbol, making one a Reiki Master.

Most Masters recommend a time lapse between the 1st and 2nd Level initiations to allow time for processing the experience; most strongly recommend a much greater time lapse between the 2nd and 3rd levels to allow time for thorough processing of Levels 1 and 2, and for further Reiki education and development of teaching skills.

In order to be successfully initiated into Reiki, the following conditions must be satisfied:

1. One must be initiated by an Usui Reiki Master.

2. The Master must be in the Usui lineage, able to trace one's Master's Initiation back in a direct line to Mikao Usui in much the same way as a Catholic Bishop can trace his lineage back via a line of bishops to Christ.

3. The initiation rite must be performed according to traditional procedures and with the correct symbols of the Western Classic Usui System.

If all conditions are satisfied, it is believed that Reiki power is conferred every time, irrespective of the spiritual belief system of the Master or of the Initiate.

Once a person has been initiated to Reiki, it is firmly believed that one retains the power for the rest of one's life. In this aspect, Reiki power resembles the permanent character of Christian Baptism.

Initiation or 'attunement' into 1st Level Reiki is commonly given in a two-day workshop. However, even before participants arrive at the venue, they are strongly advised to prepare for what their teachers consider a profound and life-changing experience. The psychic insertion of the Master Symbol in a 1st Level initiation is illustrated on the following page.

FIRST INITIATION FOR LEVEL 1

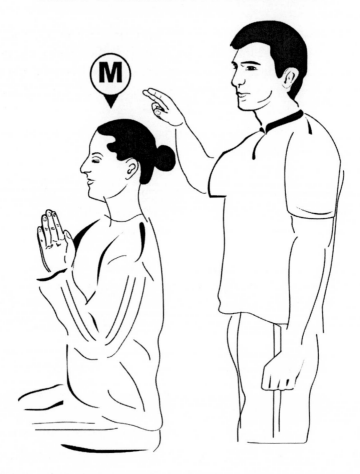

1. The Master Symbol is traced in the air over the head while the Master silently says the name (mantra) of this symbol three times. Next the Master 'guides' the symbol to the base of the head by moving the right hand down as far as the neck. Some Masters visualise the symbol drawn in the air moving into the Crown Chakra through the head and stopping at the base of the head.

The Source of Reiki

The most common name for Reiki is 'Universal Life Energy', a neutral term which makes it readily acceptable to a wide audience. Twenty years ago there was an understandable hesitation to declare its "divine" nature. Thus Eric Harz, at that time a Reiki enthusiast, wrote to Paul Mitchell, a leader of one branch of the Reiki movement: 'I wrote that I believed that the universal energy was God. He agreed, saying that Masters just do not tell people that, because Reiki would be confused by individual beliefs about God.'[16]

Today's Reiki leaders are not so coy:

Ellyard informs us: 'Reiki is an intelligent energy. Many people liken the energy to the source and all pervading power. Many traditions have a variety of names for this power, for example: God, Buddha, Mind, Nature, Universe, Great Spirit, the Force, etc.

'Regardless of semantics, essentially the importance lies in the notion that a higher force does permeate all existence and that one can tap this potential through specific methods to benefit sentient beings. What this means is that when one becomes attuned to the Reiki system, there is effectively a merging of the divinity within our own spirit with that of the creative force ... To put it simply we have a direct line to God or Buddha consciousness ... .'[17]

Frank Petter highlights Reiki's divine nature: 'Such was the greatness and genius of Dr. Usui: the ability to channel the divine into a form that can be experienced and practised by his fellow human beings.'[18]

The consensus in the Reiki world is that the Reiki source is the Divine Absolute. The label given to this supreme deity is irrelevant. Orthodox Christians have an entirely different perspective.

Spirituality without Religion

Increasingly, Reiki leaders are stressing the importance of Reiki as a source of spiritual development. For some, this spirituality emerges directly from a Reiki experience, as in the case of Klaudia Hochhuth,

one of the Reiki pioneers in Australia, who recalled her initiation into
Reiki II:

> During the initiation in the second-degree class something
> happened to me which I would describe as a reawakening or
> reconnecting with my Holy Self. For a few moments I had a
> sense of oneness with everything and everyone – a unique and
> overwhelming experience which I will never forget. It changed my
> whole life and triggered my further spiritual direction.[19]

The direction in which her 'Holy Self' led her was the passionate
embracing of the New Age Bible, 'A Course in Miracles.'

Internationally, one of the most influential leaders of the Reiki
movement, Walter Lubeck, highlights the value of discovering
'god' without religion: *Reiki offers us a personal encounter with the divine
– independent of any church, sect or holy writing.*[20] **This encounter, he
says, can only be achieved by 'those who are truly willing to
look into the clear mirror of the divine self'**[21] by Eastern forms
of meditation.

The prophets of the Reiki movement are looking well beyond
personal spiritual development. With the rapid spread of Reiki across
the globe, they see this 'dynamic spiritual power' as the means of
uniting peoples of different cultures and religions.

William Lee Rand, a US Reiki leader preaches with messianic
fervour:

> Because Reiki is spiritual, yet not a religion, it has attracted
> students from all religious and spiritual backgrounds. Catholic
> priests and nuns practise Reiki. Jews, Protestants, Muslims, Hindus
> and Buddhists practise Reiki. Jains, Zoroastrinists, Taoists, and
> Shintoists practise Reiki. Wiccans, shamans, native peoples and
> those on independent spiritual paths practise Reiki. Those in
> virtually all religious groups are attracted to the practice of Reiki.
> **An important reason is that Reiki gives each person a more
> immediate experience of the divine.** Reiki places everyone

more directly in contact with the higher power (regardless of the name one may call it) and provides direct experience of the higher power's grace and compassion. Reiki is thus helping to unite all people of the world regardless of religious or ethnic background ... the fact that Reiki can and is being sent at a distance by many people to heal world crisis situations adds another dimension to the healing Reiki provides. (emphasis added)

Rand foresees that *a critical point will be reached when there will be so much Reiki flowing on the planet that world peace will come very quickly.*[22]

10

Reiki Wreckage

A s society rapidly gives its stamp of approval to this complementary form of healing, its leaders claim that 'Reiki is guided by the higher power, it cannot do harm and always works for the positive benefit of the client'.[1] Such statements, unfortunately, are accepted by a society desperately searching for answers. The following personal accounts attest, however, that Reiki may cause great emotional and spiritual harm.

Eric Harz, a happily married man with four children, suddenly found himself in a mid-life crisis. Not only did the seductive power of Reiki bring this Spirit-filled Christian to the verge of adultery, it brought him for seven years into the practice of idolatry. What exposed the spiritual softness in Eric was a chance encounter with an old teenage friend who was visiting the USA from Germany. Suffering from a sore back, Eric asked Susie if she would give him a back massage. He got more than he bargained for:

> At one point in the massage of my lower back she spread her thumbs from the middle of my back out to my sides. With this motion an energy rushed in that quickly spread up and down my body, covering me to the top of my head, to the tips of my fingers, and to the tips of my toes. It was seductive far beyond the sexual. Susie's massage was my doorway into Reiki, my true initiation. My adulterous lust was the key that opened the door for the demon spirit of Reiki to enter. For the days immediately succeeding my whole body chemistry changed. Every excrement changed in odour, texture and/or colour: sweat, urine, faeces and even semen.

127

> I also found the lust for more power began to work within me. I
> found myself ready to take off anywhere with this woman, all to
> keep this new overwhelming energy.[2]

It was not till months later that Susie told Eric that she had given
him Reiki during the massage. So overpowering was this experience
that Eric spent the next seven years in pursuit of this energy. Or
was it rather that Reiki was pursuing Eric? His next overwhelming
experience came totally unsolicited, not from an attractive female
friend but from 'out there':

> One summer's day I 'received' a Reiki symbol. I was sunbathing at
> the pool, and although I had my eyes closed, I saw it come straight
> at me. (It had within it a cross and stick figure of a house. I knew
> such a thing was possible, because Dr. Usui, Reiki's founder, had
> himself received the Reiki symbols in a similar fashion. I sketched
> the symbol quickly and sent it to Susie to say 'what is it?'[3]

It turned out to be the Long Distance Symbol. Without going
through the standard initiation procedures from a Reiki Master, Eric
found himself with all the Reiki powers of a Level 2 graduate. This was
to lead him on a long journey into the world of Reiki, during which
he formalised his Level 1 and 2 qualifications and sought the Master's
Level through the Reiki Alliance, an international group promoting
Usui Reiki. As time went on, he began to find a growing conflict
between his Reiki energy and his walk in the Holy Spirit, between
the values espoused by Reiki people and Christian teaching, between
Reiki healing and biblical healing. Having decided to exit Reiki, he
was convinced that Reiki power is demonic power. The full story is
contained in Eric's booklet, *The Reiki Danger: Healing that Harms*.

Eric's account provides important insights into the Reiki culture,
what I summarise as:

1. The Lust Syndrome.
2. The Denial of Evil Syndrome.
3. The Anti-Christian Syndrome.

The seductive aspect of Reiki is a recurring theme in Harz's book. The overpowering effect of Susie's massage led to a prolonged relationship by phone and letter between them in different countries. Harz's deepest desire was to receive initiations into Levels 1 and 2 from Susie. However, as Susie was not a Reiki Master, this was impossible. Nor did Susie reciprocate Eric's passion. Eventually, Eric's wife Michele had a showdown with her husband, giving him a choice – Susie or her. After an agonising struggle, Eric finally opted for his wife. However, Eric was far from out of the woods. He went on to do Level 1 with Gwendolyn, who was later to become President of Reiki Alliance. Eric recalled:

> Gwendolyn was as captivating as Susie, and as seductive. The same spirit was present. Though Gwendolyn was of a different ethnic background and I had no history with her, it was that allure that had me ready to yield to her as I would have to Susie. Gwendolyn knew she had it. She even fed into it with some signs of affection during the exchange of a Reiki treatment but she seemed clearly uninterested in anything more than a teacher/student relationship.[4]

Later, Eric did Level 2 with Irene, the secretary to Paul Mitchell who was later to become joint-leader of Reiki Alliance. Again the pattern was similar, with Eric finding that Irene possessed the same seductiveness characteristic of Susie and Gwendolyn. When Eric finally became a Reiki Practitioner, he was to discover the same seductive quality within himself! In a frank appraisal he tells us:

> Later I saw the sexually seductive side of Reiki in my own work. To those who were susceptible, it was a definite side effect, and although this aspect was largely kept hidden, it worked to encourage lust in me. I found that without even trying, I encouraged lust in others. My wife's married friend told her after a healing session that if Michele weren't such a good friend, she would have had sex with me. Understand clearly that I made no conscious advances. This seductiveness is built into Reiki, and is a powerful hook. With

this type of seduction the energy has destroyed ministries and marriages.[5]

The Denial of Evil Syndrome

One of the earliest lessons Eric learned from Susie, was 'to fear nothing, to just be open to whatever came.'[6] When Susie went to India to pay homage to Sai Baba, she sent three gifts to Eric – a grey ash, vibuti, which allegedly has great powers of healing and which Baba produced 'miraculously' from his hand; a perfumed oil which appeared 'miraculously' on Baba's wrist; and a picture of Sai Baba. She wrote a note with each gift – 'fear nothing and you will not be harmed.'[7] Such an attitude leaves one naively open to the forces of evil and was the result of the Reiki culture's denial of the existence of evil.

Sometimes Reiki people went to extraordinary lengths to destroy their consciences. Eric's second teacher, Gwendolyn, tried to remove all guilt from her life. She told him:

> ... of a man with a different energy practice. Upon entering his office he had her sit in a chair across the room. He asked what she was seeking. She told him she sought to be free of the duality of right and wrong, good and bad, really seeking to be free of guilt. He moved his hands; as he did, her spirit rose up out of her body. He set the body on visible 'spirit fire'. As the fire diminished, he put her spirit back into the body. Since that time she began to believe that there was no evil, only degrees of light. Because of these experiences, she now teaches that belief as a fact.[8]

The Anti-Christian Syndrome

Reiki people warmly welcome those of all faiths and they may even embrace the comfortable parts of Christianity into the Reiki belief system. However, there are two key factors in Reiki which essentially undermine Christian faith. The first is the demonic power which is

Reiki. Harz puts it well:

> At every turn it was clear that you needed to let go of your beliefs
> to gain understanding and grow in this energy. If you carried your
> own personal faith, that was acceptable. The energy would lead
> you deeper until you let go of that conviction too, until you too
> came to their mystical, nebulous thing called 'oneness', if not in
> this life, then in another life. They said all paths lead to God.[9]

The second factor which undermines a Christian's faith is the Reiki
belief that there is no evil. Eric outlined the journey from immorality
through scepticism to disbelief:

> A big part of their teaching was that there is no evil, that 'sin' is
> a lie to bring about fear and cause us to wander from our path.
> The step from doubting sin to doubting Jesus' mission was easy.
> Without the conviction of sin, salvation offered in Jesus' name
> made no sense. Damnation had no reality for me. With no ultimate
> penalty, who would have need of a Saviour? This faulty reasoning
> all started with the premise that the scripture lacked some greater
> truth and all of Reiki is built to promote that belief.[10]

After some years in Reiki, Eric's faith in Christ had diminished: '…
by this time I was sharing a watered-down Gospel that I myself had
come to doubt. My beliefs were disjointed, and in my heart I knew
more conflict than consistency.'[11]

Towards the end of his time in Reiki, Eric began to have
reservations. These came to a head when he was shaken by a wise
servant of God who challenged him: 'It's still not Biblical healing.
Look at the Scriptures again'.[12] Eric went to the Bible and began to
study biblical healing closely. Over months, the Holy Spirit brought
him to a state of deep repentance. He concluded:

> I finally came to the point of recognising that it was a demon
> I had received during that massage. By that demon I had been
> empowered. By that demon I worked and spread my practice of

Reiki. I wanted to be clean again. I wanted to know the Holy Spirit alone at work in my life. I begged to be clean of the influences left behind... Most certainly that cleansing did come after hours, days and weeks begging the Lord. The process of inner cleansing, or sanctification, has continued even through the writing of this book, although the presence of the Reiki demon was gone from the time of my repentance.[13]

I strongly encourage any Christian involved in Reiki to read Eric's book reflectively. You too may come to perceive Reiki as the healing that harms.

Counterfeit[14] Healing

After interviewing Ruth on her involvement with Reiki I invited her to write her story for this book.

Ruth:

I was a married woman with a family of three young children living in a small country town in Victoria. I went along with my friend to do a Level 1 in a weekend workshop which took place in the home of the Reiki Master, Julie. She was a woman of about forty years and had such a beautiful presence and was very warm. Her intention was to initiate the eight of us in Level 1 first, and then in a later weekend workshop, to initiate us into Level 2. Julie started off by introducing us to the Reiki system. We were told that the founder of it was a Japanese man by the name of Usui. We were led to believe that Usui was a Christian who had based his healing Reiki on Jesus' healings.

Julie initiated us into Level 1 by going around each one of us individually and placing certain symbols on us. We did not see the symbols. Then after our initiation, we were given two symbols and told never to show them to anyone unless they were Reiki people. We were also shown the different energy centres or chakras in the human body. We were informed that each energy centre vibrated a particular colour and you experienced that colour when you had a healing through that chakra. For example, if someone was having Reiki work done on the heart, that person would see a pink colour. We were shown what organs were affected by what chakra and were shown how to lay hands on the body. After being initiated and instructed, we practised on each other. For some reason it was very exciting. I saw colour change and swirl when people moved their hands across my body. We were told to place our hands daily on the chakras in our own body as a form of self-healing. I never remember Jesus being mentioned once in these sessions, though later when we did Level 2, they did talk a lot about spirit.

We all went away to practise on each other, and then we used to get together often outside the formal sessions. A real bond began to grow amongst us and it felt like we were in a family together. We gave each other much support for all sorts of problems in our lives.

Then we moved on to do Level 2. This time we were given an additional symbol – the Long Distance Symbol. And we were now shown how to use all three symbols in our Reiki. We were taught how to send distance healing. We used a pillow as a surrogate person and we sent energy as a group and then individually to a particular person who could then give us feedback. All the feedback we received seemed positive. As the result of our Reiki, some people slept more peacefully or told us that they felt the healings to their confidence grew and we thought we were doing some good work.

Then as a group we continued to meet and practise our Reiki on people who came to us for healing. Because we met in our own homes so often, we became very close to each other and to those we worked on. Most of us were housewives with children and I guess we felt a sense of self-esteem doing this sort of work. It was an ego boost. Then one day a friend of mine named Rex, who had just become a Master, gave me a Reiki healing. I went screaming into another dimension. I was in a revolution with cannons and explosions everywhere and I was fighting for my life with soldiers using swords. I had no awareness of lying on the bed but I was in a real fight for my life in a dimension that was earthly. Those around me all realised my distress as I kicked and fought them as they used massage and crystal healing to bring me back. That was extremely scary. I don't know why I didn't just discontinue then. As I look back on it, I realise that Rex had an amazingly big ego. I vowed I would never have him give me Reiki again.

As we continued we were told that there were spirits attached to Reiki and that you could call on them and receive your own personal spirit (your Reiki spirit) to help you with the person you were working on. With the help of my Reiki spirit, I could sometimes actually see into the body and see the problem, and at other times I would know what was emotionally wrong with the person. Through my spirit, I developed a real clairvoyance. Now I really thought I could be of great help. Even though Jesus was never mentioned, I realised that some of these people were not Christians and so I kept my faith to myself. I always called upon Jesus before I healed people and I thought I sensed his presence when I was healing.

I met so many people in Reiki and they were all involved in many different New Age practices e.g., crystal healing, Tarot Cards, astrology, Past Life Regression Therapy, clairvoyance, aura drawings and healing. So the natural progression for me using my "gift", was channelling, a form of clairvoyance. It developed so quickly and naturally through Reiki that I didn't question it. Through it I became very popular and people would even come from interstate to consult me. I remember I had only one person question what I said to her. So, feeling very hurt, I gave her money back to her, at the same time telling her that she would understand when all the things I predicted came to pass. But all the other people I spoke with were amazed at what they heard.

I heard of Catholic nuns in America who ran Reiki healing centres. I even had a Catholic priest come to me for Reiki and he was interested in practising it himself. So I thought it was okay and I never questioned it.

In the meantime I experienced many different types of healing from others – crystal healing, sound healing, Past Life Regression. I developed an ability to see auras and I used that in my healings. This became a real party trick as my hand would just draw the auras spontaneously and the colours would just appear. I was very popular and you can imagine how that affected my self-esteem. All of a sudden I was not just a mum – I was someone, and that need to heal others kept getting stronger and stronger.

Then I used to attend a mediating meeting of Reiki Masters once a month. This group had requested me to channel messages from the spirit world for them. It was like being a medium at a séance. As these were all Masters, I felt very privileged to be asked. One day I channelled this being called Qwan Yin. As she entered me, my whole body shook. It was a strange phenomenon. It took a lot out of me. She was some divine goddess and I don't remember what she said. I really never remembered what these spirits said through me, but all of the Masters wanted more of this goddess so I channelled her quite a lot. I realised after a while that this sort of thing was not good for my body. So, since I was regularly in contact with my spirit-guide, I received instructions from it not to do this anymore. In fact, I was told not to channel any other spirits except one called Shannon who was particularly chosen for me to keep my mind and body safe. So we developed an incredible relationship with this spirit called Shannon and my whole family came to know him very well and listened to him.

Looking back, it all seems kind of strange, but everyone was doing the same thing so it just seemed natural. I still continued to go to church on a Sunday, enjoyed being there, and I still prayed, but there was an extra spirit-dimension to it now and I didn't question it.

At that time, like all my Reiki friends, I believed that we all had past lives. So I did a week of Past Life Regression therapy. They said that I had so much psychic debris from my past lives that I had to do this course to clear myself. So I went screaming into every session which were so violent that my physical body just shook itself. I felt exhausted after every session, and being so gullible, I believed I was on the right track.

I had many other amazing supernatural experiences. I seemed to be the one in our Reiki group that felt the most and saw the most. My following grew and I became very popular. I remember once doing a Psychic Market and having queues of people lined up for me for channelling. I did not charge them – payment was by donation only. I worked the whole day without a break and at the end of the day there were people cursing me because I didn't have time to treat them. Those were the days of stupidity, I can see now, but I thought I was giving myself to others and doing the best I could to help.

I did a weekend on Astral Travelling and found that I could actually travel to places and see into people's homes. This was very fascinating because everyone would tell me that I must have been actually there, so much was I able to tell them about their homes. I used this practice quite regularly.

I remember once being so much in the spirit that one morning I got up off the bed and I actually floated across the room until I realised what was happening, then I landed with a jolt. My spirit had not woken up!

I went for a trip overseas. While on the boat I saw the White Cliffs of Dover, and I had vision after vision of troops coming home from the war and I became convinced that there was such a thing as past lives. This type of thing happened to me all the time.

Unfortunately my whole family was involved and they all believe in past lives as well.

Because he was so impressed by my experiences, my husband did Reiki Level I. He developed a deep connection to the Reiki Master Julie. He really liked her. He never got involved as I did thank goodness. He said that when he was being initiated he saw Jesus Christ. He was so awed by this that he has never let go of this vision. I am steadily trying to tell him of the dangers of Reiki. I believe he has not given up on Reiki completely even though he does not practise anymore.

By this stage my marriage was not going well. We had a lot of problems and I had met a lovely man with whom I became friends. I remember the first time I did Reiki on him, and after that our friendship changed into something deeper, and then we had an affair. I finally left my husband for this man who never promised to commit to me. This was a terrible time for me. I had such a lot of guilt. My two boys would not come with me but stayed with my husband. I had my little girl with me. I used to go back every morning at 7.00 am and get the boys off to school and be there when they come home from school and then go back again at night. This went on for six months when I found out my boyfriend was having other women.

This put a stop to our affair and I went into counselling and great distress. I felt ripped in half and in my agony one morning I was given a divine healing – in a moment all indecision left me and I felt myself so joyful that I rang my husband and went immediately back to him.

Then one day the crunch came. A friend of mine came to me to receive Reiki from me. After the Reiki session she told me that this practice was not of God. She was a deep Christian, a fundamentalist. She absolutely devastated me and I didn't believe her. I thought she was not right, but her comment sowed a seed of doubt in my mind and I really started to pray about it. I became so distressed that we finally moved away from the area. I continued to spend much time in prayer in the local church but still could not get a sense of whether my friend was right or not. Looking back, what I think was keeping me in a state of confusion was that I was still heavily into Reiki while I was trying to work out whether it was of God or not. That's not a good mix.

Eventually the doubts and frustration made me realise that all this feeling was not of God, so I made a decision – if there was any doubt of its rightness, I should just put it behind me. And I did just that. I ripped up all my Reiki stuff and threw it away.

Shortly after this we moved interstate to Perth. It was here I met a parent at the local school, a lovely woman to whom I was immediately drawn. It turned out that she was the wife of the pastor of a local Pentecostal Church. Even though I was a Catholic, I decided to attend this Church. When in casual conversation I told the pastor's wife that I had been involved in Reiki, she said to me one explosive word – 'Counterfeit!' This word went straight to my heart and tore away the veil surrounding it. I knew instantly that Reiki was truly a counterfeit of Christian healing. So I arranged a meeting with the Pastor in which I renounced Reiki and its allied psychic powers – spiritualism, astral travel, clairvoyance, belief in past lives and reincarnation. After this a group from the Church prayed over me for some time asking that God would release me from all spiritual bondage. And as well, I re-asserted my belief that Jesus Christ was my Saviour and unique Lord and I surrendered my life to Him. At some point later, I asked for and received the Baptism in the Holy Spirit then felt much better. Still, my husband was not fully convinced that Reiki was not of God as he was still clinging to his vision of Christ.

Sometime later we moved to Sydney. Here I returned to the practice of my Catholic faith. Even though my condition had improved, I was still suffering from the scars of emotional and spiritual traumas from the past and I was still being haunted by some of those spirits I had welcomed in the past.

One significant step I took at this time was to go to the Sacrament of Reconciliation and make a general confession of all my sins including my involvement in Reiki. Fortunately for me, the priest had a good understanding of Reiki and was also very compassionate. When I left his presence, I felt a great burden had been lifted. Then, thanks to a wonderful Brother of the Church and the power of the Holy Spirit, I have had many scars removed from hurts received throughout my life.

When I was a teenager, my nickname was 'Smiley' because I used to smile a lot. And just recently I'm finding I'm beginning to smile once again. And the smile is not counterfeit. For this I give all praise to God for this journey and hope others too will recognise the dangers associated with Reiki and all practices of New Age.

Christians Embrace Reiki

I also began to stumble across others who had direct experience of Reiki. There was the Christian woman who told me she had graduated in Reiki I and II many years earlier. When she had been challenged that the practice of Reiki was at odds with her Christian beliefs, she immediately retorted 'But Sister N (a Catholic nun) practises Reiki!' Since then I have discovered a number of Catholic Sisters, both here and overseas, who are Reiki practitioners.

Many lay people in Christian churches are heavily involved. Not so long ago, a friend was quietly praying in the pew of an inner-suburban Catholic church in Sydney when she became aware of two women standing not far from her. She recognised one – a pillar of the church – who appeared to be praying quietly over the other. My friend, perhaps hoping to get in on the act, approached the couple and enquired what was happening. She was told that a Reiki session was in progress, and she was asked politely to move on.

A website, *Reiki for Christians*, both justifies Christians' involvement in Reiki and strongly encourages them to do it in the name of Christ. The arguments presented are very plausible, concluding with persuasive testimonies from three committed Catholics, two of whom are Catholic Sisters while the third, a male, is a professed member of the Dominican Third Order, who presents himself as a Master of Theology accredited by the De La Salle University, Manila. He adds that he has had extensive experience in the Catholic Charismatic Renewal and signs off as: *A Roman Catholic who happens to be a Reiki Master.*

11

Rating Reiki

Reiki Enriched Spiritualism

It is a common experience in the Reiki culture that initiations at all three levels assist in the development of psychic abilities. In this respect, Steve Murray, currently one of the most popular of international Reiki teachers, has gone a step further than most Reiki Masters. He offers a form of initiation geared to opening his students to new psychic powers and strengthening existing ones. In his guidance[1], he refers to a variety of such powers including the occult abilities of fortune-telling, seeing auras, reading 'past lives' of people, reading Tarot Cards, astral travel and channelling. In fact, he devotes a complete chapter in one of his books[2] to explaining how Reiki can be used to improve one's channelling ability.

Now if channelling is clearly contrary to biblical and church teaching[3], then the Reiki which enhances it is morally wrong and is in fact an instrument of demonic influence as Eric Harz and Ruth, both former experienced practitioners of the art, have already pointed out.

Reiki Healing v Biblical Healing

Reiki healing occurs independently of the faith system of the healer and the healed. In the Christian dispensation, healing requires faith in Jesus Christ, both on the part of the person praying for the healing of another and on the part of the person seeking to be healed.

There are numerous instances in the New Testament which illustrate the importance of faith in healing. Suffice it here to take two. On one occasion when Paul was preaching to a pagan audience in Lycaonia, a dramatic healing took place: *There was a man sitting there who had never walked in his life, because his feet were crippled from birth; he was listening to Paul preaching, and Paul looked at him intently and saw that he had faith to be cured. Paul said in a loud voice, 'Get to your feet – stand up' and the cripple jumped up and began to walk.*[4]

Paul's powerful proclamation of the death and resurrection of Jesus made such an impact on this poor cripple that he immediately believed the risen Jesus could heal him. With both Paul and the cripple sharing a common faith, a marvellous healing occurred.

The importance of having faith in God in order for healing to occur, was also brought home forcefully when Jesus visited his home town, Nazareth. Here, Jesus had great difficulty healing people because of their lack of faith: *...he could work no miracle there, except that he cured a few sick people by laying his hands on them. He was amazed at their lack of faith.*[5]

Reiki people find no such hindrance to their ability to heal and would perhaps see their healing system as being superior to that of Christianity. There is another possible explanation – the source and nature of the Reiki healing power could be different from that of Christianity.

Reiki provides healing power to all on demand. The Christian charismatic gift of healing is bestowed only on some members of the community.

During the public life of Christ, he bestowed the gift of healing on his apostles and on 72 of his lay disciples, a sub-group. Even after the extraordinary outpouring of the Holy Spirit at Pentecost, the gift of healing was bestowed only on some as St Paul makes clear in writing to a highly gifted community at Corinth:

To one is given from the Spirit the gift of utterance expressing wisdom; to another the gift of utterance expressing knowledge in accordance with the same Spirit; to another faith, from the same Spirit; to another the gift of healing, through this one Spirit; to another, the working of miracles, to another, prophecy; to another, the power of distinguishing spirits; to one the gift of different tongues and to another the gift of interpretation of tongues. But at work in all these is one and the same Spirit, distributing them at will to each individual …

Now Christ's body is yourselves, each of you with a part to play in the whole … Are all of them [the community] apostles, or all prophets, or all teachers? Or all miracle workers? Do all have the gifts of healing?[6]

Paul is making it clear that the particular gift(s) a person receives is determined not by the will of the Christian but by the will of the Holy Spirit. Only some people receive the gift of healing so that they might make their particular contribution to the building up of the body of Christ.

In Christianity, as distinct from Reiki, the gift of healing is not on tap! Indeed, if a situation arises where the power to heal is dispensed to all those who want it, we can be sure that the origin of the gift is not the Holy Spirit but a demonic spirit.

Reiki healing is transmitted from Master to Initiate by a private ritual. In Christianity the gift of healing is bestowed in a public rite of initiation into the Christian community by the direct action of the Holy Spirit.

In the initiations into the three levels of Reiki, four symbols of Buddhist origin are psychically implanted in the Initiate while the relevant mantra is recited. As well, the Master transmits Reiki power to all the main chakras by blowing over them.

For the transmission to be fruitful, the Master must be in the Usui lineage. Hence the Reiki power is transmitted via Usui from Medicine King Buddha as Usui consistently maintained.[7] As we have noted earlier, the worship of a false god is the worship of a demon hiding behind the mask of that god. Hence the source of Usui Reiki power is demonic.

In the Christian-Catholic tradition, the gift of healing comes to some as a consequence of initiation into the community through the Sacraments of Baptism and Confirmation. The bishop/priest conferring this latter must be in the lineage of the Apostles who received their power directly from the Holy Spirit sent by Christ. Hence the source of Christian healing is the Holy Spirit.

Another point of difference is that people normally pay money to receive a Reiki initiation or to receive Reiki healing. Christian healing is a free gift of the Holy Spirit, and those so gifted do not charge for their services.

The tradition of paying for a Reiki initiation or for Reiki treatment, euphemistically called 'energy exchange', was started in the West by Mrs Takata, so that people would appreciate the value of Reiki and not take it for granted. Set fees were charged for initiations into Level I, II and Master's. The standard fee for the Master's was $10,000. Over the last decade the price has dropped markedly. But Reiki is big business, and competent Masters may earn their livelihood from it. In contrast Christian healers follow Jesus' injunction to the Apostles: **You have received without charge, give without charge.**[8]

In the New Testament there is no evidence at all of people being healed through Buddhist symbols, mantras and the placing of the hands over the various 'energy centres' of the body. There is, however, much evidence of the laying on of hands, normally on the head of the person being healed.

Reiki practitioners in dealing with Christians often give the impression that the laying on of hands in Reiki is the same as that in the Christian tradition. On one occasion Klaudia Hochhuth revealed how she persuaded an elderly lady to receive treatment:

On one occasion a woman in her late 70s asked me about 'the natural modality I practise'. I knew that her husband had been killed by the Japanese during the war, and for obvious reasons she was extremely sensitive to everything which came from Japan; in fact, she hated everything which had the slightest connection with that country. Feeling that she would benefit from Reiki, I explained to her that it is channelling energy through the laying on of hands, **similar to what Jesus did as described in the Bible.** This interpretation was quite acceptable to her, and she enjoyed the series of treatments I gave her.[9] (emphasis added)

Sometimes Reiki persons go further, making outlandish statements (as was made to Ruth) that Reiki was founded by a Catholic priest named Usui!

However, the laying on of hands in the Christian tradition is fundamentally different to that in the Reiki culture. The Jewish tradition of imparting a blessing by placing both hands on the person's head was absorbed into the apostolic tradition of healing. Jesus practised this form of blessing when performing many of his healings[10], and passed on the practice to the early church: *These are the signs that will be associated with believers … they will lay their hands on the sick and they will recover.*[11]

The practice of the Apostles of combining this laying on of hands with an anointing with oil[12] laid the foundation for a more formal approach in the early church: *Any one of you who is ill should send for the elders of the church and they must anoint the sick person with oil and pray over [lay hands on] him. The prayer of faith will save the sick person and the Lord will raise him up again. So confess your sins to one another and pray for one another to be cured.*[13]

It is worthy of note that Christian healing here takes place in an atmosphere of faith in the healing power of Christ and is accompanied by confession of sin. Those involved in the healing ministry today can vouch for the value of faith and repentance in the process of healing.

In Reiki healing no faith in Christ is required (according to Harz it is often discouraged) and no importance is attached to the confession of sin, for sin implies the existence of evil, and *all Reiki teachers deny the existence of evil.*[14]

Deviating Doctrines

Despite the fact that Reiki leaders continually proclaim that Reiki is not a religion and is therefore doctrine-free, Reiki culture shares a common belief system sharply at odds with Christian doctrines:

1. The nature of Reiki's supreme deity, Supreme Chi [Wu Chi] is essentially different from the nature of the one true God of Christianity.

2. Reiki believes creation to be pantheistic and monistic, in contrast to biblical creation.

3. Sin is non-existent in Reiki; virtue and sin are a constant theme throughout the Bible.

4. There is no place for hell in the Reiki belief system; the Bible makes it emphatically clear that there is a hell for humans who freely choose to go there. (Mt 25:41; *Catechism*, 1033-1037)

5. Reiki teaches that all humans have the capacity to become divine, the Bible teaches the only divine human was Jesus Christ, and that Christians have the capacity to become Christ-like.

6. Reiki believes in Karma based on the law of strict justice; the Bible reveals a God of justice and mercy in the person of Jesus Christ. (Rev. 14:7; Lk. 23:42-43)

7. Reiki believes in reincarnation; the Bible reveals that we have only one life on this earth. (Hb. 9:27)

8. Reiki has no place for the unique Lordship of Jesus Christ. (Acts 4:1; 1Cor. 12:3)

9. Reiki is dismissive of the redemption of the human race through the life, death and resurrection of Jesus Christ. (Jn 14:6)

Reiki Immorality

Moral behaviour common in the Reiki culture is at odds with the code of morality presented in the New Testament:

1. The deliberate blunting of one's conscience by seeking to dismiss feelings of guilt connected with sin. The teachings of Christ include, and go beyond, the Ten Commandments: 'Therefore anyone who infringes even one of the least of these commandments and teaches others to do the same will be considered the least in the kingdom of Heaven; but the person who keeps them and teaches them will be considered great in the kingdom of Heaven.'[15]

2. Marital infidelity resulting from Reiki-induced lust.

3. Forms of spiritualism, fostered by Reiki treatment, in which the spirits of the dead, so called 'angels' and pagan deities are contacted with a view to obtaining information about the past, present and future. (See Dt. 18:10-12; Gal. 5:18-20; Col. 2:18; 2Th. 2:9-12; *Catechism*, 2115, 2116).

4. Reiki may develop and strengthen the ability to discover hidden things about people and to predict the future through astrology and use of horoscopes (see Is. 47:13-15; *Catechism*, 2116).

5. The practice of swallowing ash and drinking elixir (at the least superstition, at the worst idolatry) 'miraculously' produced by 'divine' Sai Baba in order to fortify the healing procedure of Reiki. (See Acts 8:9-25; 19:18-19; Rev. 21:8).

6. The common failure of Reiki people to discern the actions of people through a misinterpretation of Jesus' words: 'Do not judge and you shall not be judged.'[16] Jesus is here referring to judging the hidden motivation of a person or acting the part of God and passing judgment on a person's spiritual condition. It does not refer to assessing the objective morality of a person's behaviour. Hence the Christian saying: 'Love the sinner but hate the sin.' (See Mt. 16:1-4; 11-12; 23:1-7).

7. The blanket condemnation of all anger in the first Reiki principle,

overlooking the fact that there is a place for righteous anger in a healthy spiritual life as seen in Jesus' life. (See Mk. 3:1-6; 11:15-17; Mt. 23:13-23).

8. The common approval and practice of spiritually dangerous energy systems in Reiki culture, such as yoga and tai chi.

9. The growing practice in Reiki of using forms of meditation aimed at blanking the mind for extended periods, rendering people susceptible to demonic influence.

US Bishops Rate Reiki

In March 2009, the U.S. Conference of Catholic Bishops through its Committee on Doctrine, released a statement, *Guidelines for Evaluating Reiki as an Alternative Therapy*.[17] The document established:

- Reiki is not a scientific method of healing.
- Reiki healing is not Christian healing.
- Reiki healing contains elements of a religion.
- In the underlying belief system of Reiki, there are both monistic and pantheistic tendencies.

The statement points out that some forms of Reiki involve invoking spirit-guides to assist in the healing process and points out that *this introduces the further danger of exposure to malevolent forces or powers.*[18]

The document concludes with the following directives: *Since Reiki therapy is not compatible with either Christian teaching or scientific evidence, it would be inappropriate for Catholic institutions, such as Catholic health care facilities and retreat centres, or persons representing the Church, such as Catholic chaplains, to promote or to provide support for Reiki therapy.*[19]

Let us hope and pray that other national bodies of Catholic bishops will follow the US example and offer similar, long overdue guidelines not only on Reiki but also on yoga and tai chi.

Part D

The Age of Aquarius

12

New Age Fallacies

Underlying Religious Beliefs

The three energy systems – yoga, tai chi and Reiki – have much in common. They are underpinned by similar religious beliefs, all of which purport to offer a form of self-salvation and give rise to a wide range of occult powers. Their belief systems have much in common with New Age spirituality which is at serious odds with Christianity.

The New Age beliefs which mark them off from Christianity are:

- Monism
- Pantheism
- Impersonal Energy as supreme creator
- Karma and Reincarnation (not universally accepted in tai chi).

Salvation by Technique

All three energy practices offer a path to self-divinisation. This omega point is characteristically New Age. Though the techniques vary, they have one thing in common – a form of meditation/initiation which creates a void in the mind, an altered state of consciousness. In yoga and tai chi, years of hard work are required to master such forms of meditation. Reiki is different. No ability to meditate is required to receive any of the initiations. This is what makes this practice so attractive – power without effort, a kind of lazy person's spirituality. After initiation, channelling Reiki facilitates an A.S.C. which is highly conducive to the practice of Eastern forms of meditation such as ghasso, yoga and zen. Increasing numbers of Reiki Masters are adopting such forms of meditation to give 'bite' to their healing powers.

It seems to me that the advent of yoga and tai chi to the West has prepared the way for the later arrival of Reiki. Today, many Reiki Masters have one or both of these practices as a foundation for their Reiki. To paraphrase a scriptural passage: And now there remain these three – yoga, tai chi and Reiki, and, I suspect, the most dangerous of these is Reiki, because, without effort, it enables one through initiation, to make immediate contact with the demonic.

The Christian Perspective

In contrast to the New Age concepts of an impersonal energy and salvation by technique, Christian salvation comes through faith in the passion, death and resurrection of Jesus Christ and is developed through a direct personal relationship with God and people. The Vatican document on New Age expresses this well:

> In Christianity, salvation is not an experience of self, a meditative and intuitive dwelling within oneself, but much more the forgiveness of sin, being lifted out of profound ambivalences within oneself and the calming of nature by the gift of communion with a loving God. The way to salvation is not found simply in a self-induced transformation of consciousness, but in a liberation from sin and its consequences which then lead us to struggle against sin in ourselves and in the society around us. It necessarily moves us toward loving solidarity with our neighbour in need.[1]

Sweet Poison

In a recent address Bishop Fabian Bruskewitz made an interesting point:

> In Nebraska where I come from, at this time of the year, harvest time, there are a lot of rodents who try to intrude themselves in,

feasting on the corn, soybeans, and other products of the fields. This requires the farmers to put out appropriate amounts of rat poison to prevent this from happening. The rat poison that is put out is always 95% healthy, good, wholesome food. It is only the 5% in the poison that does the killing.[2]

This point is often overlooked by Christians readily rushing to embrace energy systems which appear to have so much genuine value. In focusing on these elements, **they fail to detect the poisons which have been so cleverly masked – the poisons of occultic meditation and idolatry**. As Fulton Sheen once said: *Most poisons are quite sweet to the lips. It is only when they are ingested that they destroy one.*[3]

CONCLUSION

There may be some who, after reading this book, become convicted of their involvement in yoga, tai chi, Reiki or some other New Age practices. It is important for such to repent before God and renounce any future involvement in such practices. Some may opt to do this privately, but it is often of much more value to seek out a mentor from your particular Christian tradition. Such a guide should be one who is a mature Christian who manifests the fruits of the Spirit (see Gal 5: 22-23), and who is also familiar with the pitfalls of New Age. It may be in the presence of the mentor or some appropriate person(s) within the church that confession and repentance of sin may occur. St. James exhorts Christians to *confess your sins to one another and pray for one another to be cured.* (Js 5:16) For those affiliated with the Catholic tradition, these words are interpreted as a recommendation to participate in the Sacrament of Reconciliation (Confession).

Reconciliation with our loving Father, important as it is, is but the first step on the journey of renewed Christian transformation. For ex-New-Agers who are re-joining a Christian church, I recommend participating in a renewal course such as a Cursillo, an Alpha Course, or a Life in the Spirit Seminar (Charismatic Renewal), an outline of each of which is presented in the glossary. Such programmes are designed to lead one to accept Jesus Christ as Saviour and Lord and to open oneself more fully to the power and gifts of the Holy Spirit, all of which provide a solid foundation for a life of prayer.

People coming out of New Age to Christianity generally have a great hunger for God. It is important that this hunger be satisfied by a strong devotional life based primarily on the word of God. Chewing the cud of God's word should become second nature. In this respect, a good mentor can be invaluable in directing one to pastures of rich spiritual nourishment. In the Catholic tradition, there is much available on different approaches to spirituality and different ways of meditating on the word of God and the life of Jesus. In this tradition, one very simple and effective way of drawing close to Jesus is by meditating on His life through the Rosary, a practice strongly endorsed by the Church. And for those who have once been involved in the occult, the Rosary is especially powerful in delivering one from demonic influence.

Finally, for those who are missing the physical fitness which yoga brings, may I recommend a regular tuning in to the DVD *Praise Moves,* through which not only will participants get all the physical benefits of yoga but will also experience a relaxed time in the presence of God absorbing His word, verifying by their own experience St Paul's words: *For you were brought at a price; therefore glorify God in your body and in your spirit which are God's.* (1Cor. 6:20)

ENDNOTES

Preface

1. Pontifical Council for Culture & Pontifical Council for Interreligious Dialogue, *Jesus Christ the Bearer of the Water of Life – A Christian Reflection on 'New Age'*, St Paul's Publications, 2002. (subsequently abbreviated to 'Water of Life')

2. In Reiki such altered states commonly occur in the process of giving Reiki to oneself or to others.

3. Lk 15: 11-32

4. St Faustina, *Divine Mercy in My Soul, Diary of St Maria Faustina Kowalska*, Divine Mercy Publications, Australia, 2005. Catholics are not obliged to accept private revelation as true. However, the devotional life of the Church has been heavily influenced by certain revelations, especially to saints. As the *Catechism of the Catholic Church* states (67): 'Guided by the magisterium of the Church, the *sensus fidelium* knows how to discern and welcome in these [private] revelations whatever constitutes an authentic call of Christ or his saints to the Church.'

5. In *Water of Life* (p. 64), hypnotism is bracketed with such mind-altering techniques as sustained hyperventilation, use of a yogic mantra and transcendental meditation which all 'reproduce mystical states at will' and which 'create an atmosphere of psychic weakness (and vulnerability)'. It is worthy of note that it is common practice for channellers to use hypnosis as a means of facilitating the occult practice of contacting their spirit-guides.

6. Aldous Huxley, a patriarch of New Age, regularly took mescaline and on his deathbed took LSD while his wife read passages from the Tibetan Book of the Dead which deals with the experience between the point of death and one's supposed next reincarnation. Stan Grof, a leader in New Age and a trend-setter in experimenting with non-ordinary states of consciousness, claims to have conducted 4,000 sessions of psychedelic therapy using drugs.

7. John Ankerberg & John Weldon, *Encyclopedia of New Age Beliefs*, Harvest House Publishers, Oregon, 1996. (subsequently abbreviated to E.N.A.B.), pp. 17-25

8. E.N.A.B., p. 20

9. Malachi Martin, *Hostage to the Devil*, Readers Digest Press, 1976, p. 403

10. Ibid., p. 404

11. Jn 19:34

1: Out of India

1. J.M. Dechanet O.S.B., *Christian Yoga*, Search Press, 1978, p. 54

2. Rabrindranath R. Maharaj, *Death of a Guru*, Hodder & Stoughton, 1986, p. 207

3. Gopi Krishna, *Kundalini: The Evolutionary Energy of Man*, Shambhala Publications Inc., 1997, Chapter 4

4. E.N.A.B.. p. 253

5. For a treatment of karma and reincarnation see p. 32

6. Fred Grigg, *The Deception of Martial Arts & Yoga*, Mandate Ministries Australia, 1998, p. 23

7. E.N.A.B., p. 597

8. Stan and Christina Grof, 'Spiritual Emergencies', *Yoga Journal USA*, July-Aug., 1984, p. 40

9. Ibid. p. 41

10. E.N.A.B., p. 597

11. Ibid., p. 598

12. Editors Stan & Christina Grof, *Spiritual Emergency: When Personal Transformation Becomes a Crisis*, Penguin Putnam Inc., 1989.

13. John Ankerberg & John Weldon, *The Coming Darkness: Confronting Occult Deception*, Harvest House Publishers, Oregon, 1983

14. E.N.A.B., p. 598

15. loc.cit.

16. loc. cit.

17. loc. cit.

18. loc. cit.

19. Ibid., p. 599

20. Brenda Skyrme, *Martial Arts & Yoga, A Christian Viewpoint*, New Wine Press, 1995, p. 25

21. loc. cit.

22. Ibid., p. 26

23. *Spiritual Emergency*, op.cit., p. 229

24. *Family Watch*, Issue 15, Catholic Church Insurances Ltd, pp. 1-2.

25. loc. cit.

26. loc. cit.

2: The Philosophy of Yoga

1. E.N.A.B., p. x

2. Ibid., p. 601

3. Ibid., p. 228

4. Paramahansa Yogananda, *Autobiography of a Yogi*, Axiom Publishing, 2004, p. 221

5. Ibid., p. 222

6. Swami Vivekananda, *Raja Yoga or Conquering the Individual Nature*, Trio Process Printers, Kolkata, 2004, p. 68

7. Yogananda, op. cit., p. 16

8. Mircea Eliade, *Yoga: Immortality and Freedom*, Princeton University Press, 1990, p. 10

9. Acts 4:1

10. Ps 145:8-9

11. Lk 23:43

12. Ex 20:1, 3

13. Deepak Chopra & David Simon, *The Seven Spiritual Laws of Yoga*, Pan Macmillan Australia, 2004, p. 11

14. E.N.A.B., p. 596

15. Svatmarama, *The Hathayogapradipika*, The Adyar Library & Research Centre, Chennai, India, 2000, p. 4

16. Swami Muktananda, *Play of Consciousness*, SYDA Foundation, 2000, p. 206

17. Barbara Szandorowska, *Escape from the Guru*, Marc, 1991, p. 90

18. Mother Teresa, *Come Be My Light*, Ed. Brian Kalodiezchuk M.C., Doubleday, 2007, p. 2

19. Vivekananda, op. cit., p. 35

20. Maharaj, op. cit., pp. 157-158

3: From the Holy Spirit?

1. *Catechism of the Catholic Church*, 2116. Subsequently abbreviated to *Catechism*

2. 1 Cor 10:19-20

3. Francis MacNutt, *Deliverance from Evil Spirits*, Chosen Books, 2009, p. 114

4. loc. cit

5. loc. cit

6. Ibid., p. 115

7. Maharaj, op. cit., p. 75

8. Ibid., p. 59

9. *Catechism*, 1022

10. Phil 2:9-11

11. Maharaj, op. cit., p. 204

12. Acts 4:1

13. Maharaj, op. cit., p. 206

14. *Australian Yoga Life*, op. cit., p. 63

15. Tal Brooke, *Riders of the Cosmic Circuit*, Albatross Books, 1986, p. 62

16. Ibid., p. 63

17. *Riders of the Cosmic Circuit*, p. 169

18. Ibid., p. 171

19. Gn 1:31

20. Gn 1:28

21. *Catechism*, 405

22. Ibid., 400

23. Ibid., 409

24. 1Cor. 10:31

25. St John Baptist de la Salle, *A Collection of Various Short Treatises for the use of the Brothers of the Christian Schools*, trans. W.J. Battersby fsc, Lasallian Publications Christian Brothers Conference, Maryland USA, 1993, p. 78

4: Monkeying with Minds in the Monastery

1. I have not included a treatment of Dechanet's so-called Christian Yoga in this book. I critique it in my as yet unpublished manuscript, *Yoga, Tai Chi & Reiki: A guide for Christian Leaders*. With the highest of motives, Dechanet successfully divorces his yoga from its Hindu religious belief system. The fatal flaw in his approach is that he retains two techniques which result in an altered state of consciousness: retarded breathing and a raja yoga technique of concentration. He embraced the practice of Kundalini Yoga together with the occult psychic powers which accompany it. Later in life, he became obsessed with the practice of astrology.

2. Bede Griffiths, *The One Light: Bede Griffith's Principal Writings*, ed. Bruno Barnhart, Templegate Publishers, 2001, p. 372

3. Shirley du Boulay, *Beyond the Darkness: A Biography of Bede Griffiths*, Random House, 1998, p. 138

4. Griffiths, op. cit., p. 277

5. Ibid., p. 276

6. Ibid., p. 460

7. Ibid., p. 187

8. Du Boulay, op.cit., p. 149

9. Pat Means, *The Mystical Maze, Campus Crusade for Christ*, 1976; www.amcbryan. btinternet.co.uk; TM: *Hinduism in a Scientist's Smock*, p. 1, 10; Du Boulay, op.cit., p. 172

11. Means, op.cit., p. 2

12. loc. cit.

13. loc. cit.

14. Ibid., p. 1.

15. Cardinal Jame Sin, *Pastoral Statement on certain doctrinal aspects of the Maharishi Technology of the Unified Field*, 1984. Full text available online.

16. See p. 25

17. Means, op. cit., p. 4

18. Congregation for the Doctrine of the Faith, *On Some Aspects of Christian Meditation*, 1989, online, op.cit., No. 7

19. Merv Fowler, *Zen Buddhism: Beliefs and Practices*, Sussex Academic Press, 2005, p. 109

20. Ibid., p. 125

21. Thomas Merton, *Mystics and Zen Masters*, Delta Publishing, 1967, p. 209

22. *Declaration on the Relations of the Church to Non-Christian Religions*, No. 2

23. William H. Shannon, *Thomas Merton: An Introduction*, St Anthony Messenger Press, 2005, p. 116

24. loc. cit.

25. Jung's 'Therapeutic Yoga', endowed with the psychological name 'Active Imagination', is critiqued in my as yet unpublished *Yoga, Tai Chi & Reiki: A Guide for Christian Leaders*. Jung privately claimed that this therapy was a Westernised form of Kundalini Yoga by means of which he himself had become divinised as the Aryan Christ.

26. Hesse for a time received therapy from the Jungist therapist Josef Laing and from Jung himself. It was during his short conversion to the Jungist cult that he wrote the novel *Demian* which captured brilliantly the essence of Jungism and thus popularised New Age values long before they became fashionable.

27. Sri Aurobindo's yogic philosophy was greatly admired and followed by Bede Griffiths whose naivete in this respect is treated in the manuscript mentioned in note 25.

28. Marilyn Ferguson, *The Aquarian Conspiracy: Personal and Social Transformation in the 1980s*, Granada Publishing, 1984, p. 462

29. *On Some Aspects of Christian Meditation*, No. 12

30. Ibid., footnote 12

31. M.Basilea Schlink, Pamphlet, *Christians, Yoga & TM, Evangelical Sisterhood of Mary*, Theresa Park, NSW, 1975, p. 13

32. Anne Simpson, 'Resting in God: An Interiew with Fr. Thomas Keating', *Common Boundary*, Sept./Oct. 1997, p. 5

33. Thomas Keating, *Open Mind, Open Heart*, Amity, N.Y., 1986, p. 114

34. Ibid., p. 127

35. *Integral Contemplative Christianity*, Video Series, Clip No. 17

36. M. Basil Pennington, *Awake in the Spirit*, St. Paul Publications, Middlegreen U.K., p. 94

37. Ps. 70:1

38. *John Cassian Conferences*, trans. Colm Luibheid, Paulist Press, 1985, pp. 133, 140

39. *The Cloud of Unknowing and the Book of Privy Counselling* , ed. William Johnston, Image Books, 1973, p. 92

40. *The Collected Works of St. Teresa of Avila*, trans. Kieran Kavanaugh O.C.D. & Otilio Rodriguez O.C.D., I.C.S Publications, 1980, Vol. 2, pp. 325-326

41. Ibid., Vol. 1, p. 121

42. *On Some Aspects of Christian Meditation*, op.cit., footnote 12

43. Father John Dreher, *The Danger of Centring Prayer*, www.saint-mike.org/warfare/library/wp-content/docs/ce…, p. 1

44. loc. cit.

45. *Open Mind, Open Heart*, p. 120

46. Dreher, op. cit., p. 3

47. loc. cit.

48. Ibid., p. 2

49. *Open Mind, Open Heart*, p. 37

50. Simpson, op.cit., p. 4

51. Philip St. Romain, *Kundalini Energy and Christian Spirituality: A Pathway to Growth and Healing*, The Crossroad Publishing Company, Foreword

52. Johnette S. Benkovic, *The New Age Counterfeit*, Queenship, 1993, see pp. 21-32

53. See Chapter 13, New Age Fallacies.

5: A Genuine Christian Alternative to Yoga

1. Laurette Willis, *Praise Moves* DVD, 'The Christian Alternative to Yoga', Harvest House Publishers, Oregon USA, 2006

2. Laurette Willis, *Praise Moves Booklet*, 'The Christian Alternative to Yoga', Harvest House Publishers, Oregon USA, 2006

3. Laurette Willis, 'Why a Christian Alternative to Yoga', www.praisemoves.com

4. Ibid., p. 5

5. www.praisemoves.com

6: Just An Innocent Pastime

1. Grand Master Gary Khor, *Tai Chi Qigong: For Stress Control and Relaxation*, Simon & Schuster, 1999, p. 159

2. Angus Clark, *The Complete Illustrated Guide to Tai Chi*, Element Books Ltd, 2000, p. 57

3. Kenneth S.Cohen, *The Way of Qigong: The Art and Science of Chinese Energy Healing*, Ballantine Publishing Group, 1999, p. 35

4. Khor, op. cit., p. 40

5. E.N.A.B., p. 352

6. 'Lidcombe Catholic Club', *Yours Magazine*, Dec. 2007, p. 19

7. *Lao Tsu, Tao Te Ching*, trans. Feng & English, Vintage Books, 1989, p. 18

8. Grand Master Gary Khor, *Tai Chi Khor-Style*, p. 7

9. Lao Tsu, op. cit., p. 3

10. Brenda Skyrme, *Martial Arts & Yoga: A Christian Viewpoint*, New Wine Press, 1995, pp. 23-25

11. loc. cit.

12. loc. cit.

13. loc. cit.

14. Tony Anthony (with Angela Little), *Taming the Tiger*, Authentic Media, 2004

15. Ibid., p. 18

16. Ibid., p. 23

17. Ibid., p. 56

18. Ibid., pp. 144, 146

19. Ibid., p. 167

20. loc. cit.

21. Ibid., pp. 167-168

22. loc. cit.

23. Ibid., p. 197

24. Ibid., p. 22

25. Skyrme, op.cit., pp. 110-111

26. Wolfe Lowenthal, *There Are No Secrets*, North Atlantic Books, 1991, p. 4

27. Lowenthal, op.cit., p. 102

28. Ibid., p. 103

7: Taoist Philosophy

1. Mircea Eliade, *Shamanism: Archaic Techniques of Ecstasy*, Princeton University Press, 2004, pp. 5-6

2. Lao Tsu, op. cit., p. 51

3. Ibid., p. 6

4. Ibid., p. 16

5. Lowenthal, op. cit., p. 20

6. Lao Tsu, op. cit., see p. 17

7. Ibid., p. xii

8. Ibid., p. xxv

8: To Chi or not to Chi

1. Cohen, op. cit., p. 14

2. E.N.A.B., p. 374

3. loc. cit.

4. 1Cor 10:19-20

5. *Catechism*, 390

6. Ibid., 417

7. Ibid., 418.

8. Rom 7:15-23

9. Rom 7:24-25

10. E.N.A.B., p. 362

11. Gn 1:27-28, 31

12. Mt 22:37

13. *Illustrated Bible Dictionary*, Hodder & Stoughton, 1980, Australia, Pt. 2, p. 625

9: A Crypto-Religion

1. Walter Lubeck, *Frank Arjava Petter, William Lee Rand, The Spirit of Reiki*, Lotus Press, 2006, p. 8

2. loc. cit.

3. Klaudia Hochhuth, *Practical Guide to Reiki: an Ancient Healing Art*, Gemcraft Books, 1993, p. 140

4. Ibid., p. 47

5. loc. cit.

6. loc. cit.

7. Lawrence Ellyard, *The Tao of Reiki*, Full Circle, 2002, p. 141.

8. loc.cit.; Hochhuth, op. cit., p. 52

9. Hochhuth, op. cit., p. 47; Lubeck & others, op.cit., p. 108

10. Ellyard, op. cit., pp. 46-47

11. loc. cit.

12. Ibid., pp. 33-34

13. Ibid., pp. 202-203

14. Frank Arjava Petter, *Reiki Fire*, Lotus Press, 2005, p. 117

15. Lubeck, et al, op. cit., p. 269

16. Eric Harz, *The Reiki Danger: Healing that Harms*, Jubilee Resources, Evansville IN, USA, 2001, pp. 20-21

17. Ellyard, op. cit., p. 121

18. Lubeck & others, op. cit., p. 93.

19. Hochhuth, op. cit., p. 140

20. Lubeck & others, op. cit., p. 135

21. Ibid., p. 246

22. Ibid., pp. 269-270

10: Reiki Wreckage

1. Lubeck & others, op. cit., p. 69

2. Eric Harz, op. cit., pp. 7-8

3. Ibid., p. 9

4. Ibid., p. 13

5. Ibid., p. 27

6. Ibid., p. 9

7. loc. cit.

8. Ibid., p. 17

9. Ibid., p. 25

10. Ibid., p. 28

11. Ibid., p. 24

12. Ibid., p. 29

13. Ibid., p. 30

14. 'Counterfeit' in this sense refers to demonic deception through which humans may be deceived by the evil one into believing that Reiki healing comes from the One True God as revealed by Judeo-Christianity. That Reiki healing is demonic in nature is shown by its fruits, which is demonstrated in the life of Ruth and Eric Harz and which we explain in more detail in the following chapter.

11: Rating Reiki

1. *Reiki the Ultimate Guide*

2. Ibid.

3. Dt 18:10-11; *Catechism*, 2116, 2117

4. Acts 14:8-10

5. Mk 6:1-6

6. 1Cor. 12:8-11, 28-30

7. Ellyard, op. cit., p. 50

8. Mt 10:8

9. Hochhuth, op. cit., p. 56

10. Mk 6:5; 10:16

11. Mk 16:18

12. Mk 6:12-13

13. Js 5:14-16

14. Harz, op. cit. p. 47

15. Mt 5:17-19

16. Ibid., 7:1

17. U.S. Conference of Catholic Bishops, Committee on Doctrine, *Guidelines for Evaluating Reiki as an Alternative Therapy*, online

18. Ibid., p. 6

19. Ibid., pp. 5-6

12: New Age Fallacies

1. *Water of Life*, p. 64

2. *Fidelity*, December 2006, p.18

3. loc. cit.

GLOSSARY

Alpha Course. This 10-week informal course in basic Christianity generally commences with the group spending a week away together in which the first four units of the course are covered. Thence the meetings are weekly, each session beginning with a meal followed by a talk and small-group discussion. In this relaxed setting, people are free to raise any questions. The Course originated in an Anglican Parish in England in 1990. Since then it has mushroomed into a world-wide movement espoused by a large range of Christian denominations including the Catholic Church. It focuses on the participants' relationship with Jesus and the infilling with the Holy Spirit and the various charismatic gifts.

active imagination. A form of psychotherapy developed by Carl G. Jung and practised by his school of Analytical Psychology. It is a blend of spiritualism and a Western form of yoga, the ultimate purpose of which is to divinise the patient.

acupuncture. In traditional Chinese medicine, fine needles are inserted at specific points to stimulate, disperse and regulate the flow of chi in order to restore a healthy energy balance. Because of the occult power involved, it presents spiritual dangers to the recipients.

ASC. Altered states of consciousness in which the mental processes have been significantly reduced. Such altered states leave one susceptible to demonic influence.

astral travel. The occult power enabling the spirit to leave one's body and move through the cosmos.

ba gua (the 8 diagrams). A set of eight diagrams in the I Ching representing all possible dynamic relationships between yin and yang. Each of the eight basic moves in tai chi corresponds to one of the eight diagrams.

aura reading. The occult ability to see the aura of a person and to interpret it.

ashram. A place of retreat where one goes to study under a guru.

avatar. According to Hindu belief, the incarnation of a god in human or animal form.

bhagwan. Hindi word for god.

bliss. In Hinduism, the alleged state of perfect happiness attained when a person becomes totally one with the divine absolute and with the cosmos, i.e., reaches a state of enlightenment.

Brahman. The supreme impersonal god of Hinduism, essentially different from the supreme God of Christianity.

Buddha. Lit. 'the enlightened one', refers normally to the historical **Buddha Gautama Siddhartha** (~500 BC), the founder of Buddhism.

Buddhism. A religion based on the experience and teaching of Buddha who taught that desire brings sorrow and that the removal of desire brings peace and ultimately enlightenment leading to nirvana. Does not require a supreme deity though many sects accept one.

Centring (Centering) Prayer. (C.P.) A technique of entering into an ASC through the repetition of a sacred word. This mental void allegedly brings one into contact with the divine True Self which supposedly marks the beginning of Christian contemplation. C.P. rests upon the false assumptions that a human technique can achieve what is proper to divine grace; that part of the self is God, and that feelings of being spaced out or of bliss are evidence of contact with God.

chakra. In Hindu yoga, depots of prana within the human body.

charismatic gifts. In Christianity, spiritual gifts such as healing, prophecy, reading hearts, etc, given freely to an individual to help build up the body of Christ. Not an indicator of personal holiness.

channelling. In spiritualism, the modern term to describe the process whereby a person acting as a medium receives messages from the spirit world and conveys them to others; in Reiki, the process of receiving chi from the source and transmitting it to oneself or others for the purpose of healing.

chi (qi, ki). In Taoist philosophy, divine energy present in the cosmos, an extension of the supreme absolute deity, the Tao, often referred to as 'the source'. Similar to prana but essentially different from the Holy Spirit of Christianity.

chi kung (qigong). The art of cultivating, storing and moving chi within the human body. The active form involves physical movement as in tai chi; the passive form involves meditation in stillness. The most extreme passive form is Reiki in which chi is infused directly from the source (the Tao), through a process of initiation, thus bypassing years of disciplined practice as in other forms of chi kung.

clairvoyance. The occult power of being able to see in the supernatural realm things past, present and future.

contemplative prayer. Gazing at God with love; a gift of prayer of the heart in which by God's action the activity of the intellect is suspended.

crystals. In New Age circles, quartz crystals are commonly believed to have the power to unite people with the cosmos, based on the unscientific view that crystal vibrates at the same rate as brainwaves. Normally it is occult powers which emanate from the crystal. Crystals are often used to transmit Reiki.

Cursillo. A 3-day renewal retreat which includes 15 talks on basic Christianity given by a team of priests and laity, each followed by small-group discussion; followed up by regional weekly/monthly gatherings. Its purpose is to form Christian lay leaders who will spread Christianity in society. The Cursillo Movement originated in the Catholic Church in Spain in the 1940s and has since spread worldwide and has been adopted by some other mainline churches.

discursive prayer. A form of mental prayer in which the intellect plays a more active role than the heart; conversational prayer which may include the making of acts, e.g., of faith, adoration, thanksgiving, love.

divination. The ability to predict the future by such occult means as astrology, clairvoyance, Tarot cards, the I Ching and channelling.

darshan. The meeting of a group of disciples to receive teaching from their guru.

dualism. Perceiving reality in terms of opposites, e.g., body/soul, ego/spirit, good/evil, creature/creator, as opposed to viewing all things as one as in monism.

demonisation (demonic infestation). The inhabiting of the human body by a demon or demons to the point where one or more areas of the person may be controlled. Is relatively common. The demonised may be freed by the practice of spiritual disciplines such as prayer, fasting and (in the Catholic tradition) by the frequentation of the Sacraments, especially that of Reconciliation and the Eucharist. To be distinguished from Possession (see glossary).

ego. In popular usage, the conscious part of the personality which includes the intellect, the will and emotions. In Hindu Vedantic philosophy, is seen as illusory and in need of being destroyed. In Christianity, considered good in itself but weakened by the effects of original sin and in need of being subject to the Holy Spirit dwelling within the person.

enlightenment. In Hinduism, the point at which one attains divinity thus becoming immortal after death and breaking the cycle of reincarnation.

External Chi Healing. The healing of others through the transmission of chi by touch.

ghasso. A form of meditation which aims at emptying the mind by focusing on the tips of one's fingers while hands are joined in front of the heart in the prayer position. Used by Usui and his disciples immediately before giving Reiki to make them more open channels of chi.

guru. A teacher of yoga so spiritually advanced as to be regarded as a manifestation of Brahman.

hari (hara). The energy centre, called in Chinese medicine the tan tien, in yoga the sacral chakra, is situated just below the navel and is associated with the seat of personal power and vital life force (chi, prana).

hatha yoga. A form of yoga which places stress on physical postures and controlled breathing; may include the spiritually dangerous kundalini yoga.

inner healing. In Christian circles, the process of healing past emotional hurts through the power of the Risen Christ.

I Ching (Book of Changes). Chinese classic on Taoist philosophy as a means of divination, based on the theory of yin/yang; also influential in the development of tai chi.

Jungian. One who is interested in, and supportive of the teachings of the Analytical Psychologist Carl G. Jung.

Jungist. One who belongs to the religious cult at the core of Jung's psychology and who practices his Westernised form of Kundalini Yoga called Active Imagination.

Krishna. The most popular and loved of the Hindu gods; presumed to be one of the reincarnations of Vishnu. Well known in the West through the Hare Krishna movement whose members believe they will achieve happiness and salvation through the Hare Krishna chant.

Kali. A popular Hindu goddess, who, though fierce and violent at times, has the heart of a mother, which accounts for her many devotees. She is the kundalini within the human body.

karma. A belief common to Hinduism, Buddhism, and to a lesser and modified extent, Taoist philosophy, and to New Age, based on the view that all actions have an effect on one's present and alleged future lives. At the end of one's life, the karmic bank balance determines the nature of one's next incarnation. Each person must suffer according to a law of strict justice for their own misdeeds, as there is no divine forgiveness in karma.

Karuna Reiki. Developed by William Lee Rand on the foundation of Western Usui Reiki, it includes additional symbols and the chanting of the names of the symbols while giving Reiki. Members of this school of compassionate action (Karuna), claim it is more powerful than Usui Reiki.

kundalini. An occult practice which may be used in all forms of yoga, in tai chi and in T.M. Lit., the name of a Hindu goddess symbolised by a snake with three and a half coils, and believed by Hindus to be sleeping at the base of the human spine with its tail in its mouth. The snake is supposedly aroused from its sleep by certain yogic techniques. From another perspective, the rousing of the kundalini is viewed as the transformation of sexual energy to pranic (divine) energy which rises up the spine passing through the different chakras till it reaches the crown chakra, at which point enlightenment allegedly occurs. As the prana/serpent rises, it often produces certain occult powers called siddhis. Without proper control, the rise of the kundalini will often rage like a vicious snake within a person with irresistible force. The result may be a breakdown in health, impotence, insanity or even death.

kung-fu. A martial art commonly based on the occult power of chi.

Lao Tsu. (~300 BC). Famous Chinese sage, alleged author of the first comprehensive classic work on Taoist philosophy, the Tao Te Ching, which was influential in the development of tai chi and Reiki.

Life in the Spirit Seminar. A Catholic renewal course consisting of 7 two-hour sessions, generally conducted over 7 weeks, or occasionally on a week-end live-in. Each session comprises a talk, a small-group discussion followed by prayer. Participants prepare for each session by meditating on a set passage of scripture daily. The course aims to assist one to enter more deeply into a personal relationship with Jesus Christ, to experience the in-filling of the Holy Spirit, and to integrate both into one's Christian walk. The Seminar originated in the Word of God Community, Ann Arbor, Michigan, USA in 1971, then spreading quickly across the world through the Catholic Charismatic Movement. The Seminar has also been used within the charismatic movements of some mainline churches.

Mahavairochana. The personification of Universal Life Energy, the supreme deity of Shingon Buddhism, the religion of Mikao Usui, the founder of Reiki.

mantra. A sound of one or more syllables used in yoga to assist in inducing an altered state of consciousness. One need not know the meaning of the mantra which is normally the invocation of a spirit or deity.

martial arts. Ancient methods of self-defence many of which are based on Eastern philosophies or religions; it is these latter and/or mind-altering techniques which make them spiritually dangerous.

Master. A teacher of tai chi; in Reiki, one who has reached Level 3 and hence is able to perform initiations and give advanced teaching.

maya. The Hindu belief that Brahman is the sole reality in this world and all else is illusion. Humans commonly fail to perceive this one reality, accepting illusory forms as real. Salvation comes through enlightenment which dispels this illusion.

Medicine King Buddha. In Shingon Buddhism, the Buddha most concerned with healing in all its forms; the patron deity of Reiki.

meridians. The network of channels along which divine energy (chi) flows.

monism. The belief that all is one and one is all; the opposite to dualism.

namahste. A Hindu greeting performed with hands joined in front of the heart and a polite bow. For some, it is simply 'hello', for others, especially in yoga circles, it means, 'I salute the divine person which you are'.

New Age. A loosely structured global movement of spirituality in which monistic pantheism plays a central role and in which occult practices are common. It distances itself from orthodox Christianity.

nirvana. The Hindu and Buddhist concept of heaven. It is nothingness, the bliss that results from no longer being able to feel either pain or pleasure through the extinction of the ego by absorption into pure being.

OM (AUM). Regarded by Hindus as the most fundamental and most powerful of all mantras. Its repetition invokes all Hindu gods and makes them present within the mantrist in a powerful way.

occult. Secret, hidden; related to the demonic. It is this last meaning which is intended by the author throughout this book unless otherwise stated.

past life regression therapy. The use of hypnosis to send people back to past lives with the intention of resolving past emotional or spiritual conflicts affecting one's present life. Its apparent success in accessing past lives may be largely attributable to demonic influence operating while the patient is in a trance state.

pantheism. The belief that god is all and all is god.

Pelagianism. The doctrine taught by the monk-theologian Pelagius in the fifth century which denies the transmission of original sin and claims that humans can attain salvation by their own human effort without the necessity of grace. From a Christian perspective, yoga and tai chi are forms of Pelagianism.

possession. The inhabiting of the human body by demons to the extent of controlling the core of the human personality resulting in a compulsion to perform evil. Is relatively rare. In the Catholic

Tradition, the possessed may be freed by the Rite of Exorcism.

prana. A term used in Hindu yoga to describe divine energy; Brahman as manifested in the cosmos. In essence, a very similar reality to chi.

pundit. A Brahmin who is especially learned in Hinduism.

Quan Yin. The Chinese name of a well-known Buddhist goddess of compassion and mercy.

Qigong Shibashi. Using the active form of chi kung called tai chi, through 18 successive movements, to develop, move and store divine chi.

re-birthing breathwork. A New Age alternative therapy for treating traumas associated with childbirth; involves sustained hyperventilation for one hour inducing an ASC. This allegedly increases the prana level in the patient resulting in a release of suppressed emotions related to childbirth traumas. Both the ASC and the prana philosophy underlying this practice make it spiritually dangerous.

Reiki. A branch of chi kung which aims at healing, not through personal/cosmic chi, but through chi coming directly from the supreme divinity of Taoism, the Tao, commonly called 'the source'. It differs from all other forms of chi kung in that its healing power is obtained immediately following initiation without requiring years of disciplined practice.

Reiki initiation. A set procedure performed by a qualified Master, using sacred symbols of Buddhist origin, by which the initiate receives the occult healing power of chi.

Reiki lineage. The ability to trace one's Reiki empowerment back in an unbroken line of Masters to Usui himself who received his healing powers through the mediation of a Buddhist deity, Medicine King Buddha.

Reiki symbols. In Western Usui Reiki, the four symbols borrowed from Japanese Buddhism which are psychically implanted during the ritual of initiation. These, with their accompanying shorthand used in this book, are: power, P; mental/emotional, E; long distance, D; master, M.

Rei Jyutu Ka. A Japanese spiritualist society of which Usui was a member when he discovered Reiki.

reincarnation. In Hinduism, Buddhism and New Age, the belief that humans have many lifetimes to perfect themselves before reaching divinisation and arriving at the immortal bliss of nirvana.

sartori. Japanese Buddhist term for enlightenment.

sannyasin. An initiated disciple of a guru.

shaktipat. The touch/blessing of the guru in which occult power is transferred. This power may knock the worshipper to the ground or result in a variety of psychic experiences including the arousal of the kundalini.

Shamanism. The most primitive of religions based on the inspiration and leadership of the shaman. In ancient China, the shaman was a specialist in the 'trance-dance', during which his soul was believed to leave his body and communicate with the dead, demons and nature spirits; he generally displayed occult powers. Chinese shamans, later referred to as sages, played a key role in the origins of Taoist philosophy.

Shen Ming. Lit. 'illumined spirit'. The trance state of Chinese shamans which enabled them to make contact with the spirit world. The art of tai chi aims to produce this same state.

Shingon. A Japanese Buddhist sect to which Usui belonged, the supreme deity of which has much in common with the Tao of Taoist philosophy.

Siddha. 1. An enlightened master. 2. The power transmitted by an enlightened master through the shaktipat. 3. Siddha Yoga – the name adopted by a commercial enterprise established by Muktananda in which stress is placed on kundalini yoga and shaktipat intensives.

Sensei (pron. sense-eye). A teacher of martial arts and (in Japan) a master of Reiki.

siddhis. A term used to describe various occult powers gained through the practice of yoga.

sound healing. A practice current in some New Age circles of using certain types of music or sounds to effect a healing while the patient is in a very relaxed state.

spirit-guide. A demonic spirit which masquerades as a guardian angel, often manifesting itself to the person and giving clear, direct messages.

spiritualism (spiritism). The practice of making contact with spirit entities, be it spirits of the dead, spirit-guides, angels or pagan deities. Hiding behind the mask of such 'entities' are demonic powers.

sutra. The written teachings of a spiritual master.

swami. A yogi who belongs to a particular Hindu religious order characterised by celibacy.

swamiji. A revered swami.

Tai Chi. When written as shown with capital letters in this book, the Taoist philosophical concept manifested when the Great Void (Wu Chi) becomes converted into motion (yang) perfectly balanced by stillness (yin).

tai chi. As used in this book without capital letters, the disciplined practice of sets of exercises with flowing, graceful movements accompanied by meditation, and strongly influenced by the concepts of yin and yang.

Takata (Mrs). A Japanese-Hawaiian woman who brought a modified form of Usui Reiki from Japan to the West; regarded as the matriarch of Western Reiki; responsible for spreading a highly distorted picture of the origins of Reiki and of Usui's religious beliefs.

tan tien. In tai chi and Chinese medicine, a major energy centre a few cm below the navel; the most important storage centre for chi in the body.

Tantra. A school of yoga that uses disciplines of sensual pleasure, esp. sexual experience, to attain spiritual enlightenment. Kundalini yoga emerged from this school.

Tantra of the Lightning Flash. A Buddhist text, allegedly dating back to the time of the Buddha, which contains esoteric techniques of healing, upon which Usui relied in developing his modernised form of such healing known as Reiki.

Taoism (pron. dow-ism). 1. A Chinese philosophy which is in essence a system of religious beliefs, at the core of which is a supreme deity, the Tao; based on shamanic revelations and the observation of nature; teaches that the essence of all created things is divine chi, which is composed of complementary opposites, yin and yang; is a form of pantheistic monism. 2. The religion which is derived from this philosophy.

Tao Te Ching (pron. dow day ching). The Chinese classic work on Taoist philosophy, regarded as the 'bible' of both the philosophy and the religion; a major influence on the development of tai chi.

Tarot cards. A pack of seventy-eight cards used to provide occult insights about someone's personality and future. The person picks out cards from the pack and the reader interprets their meaning.

Tibetan Reiki. A form of Reiki based on Western Usui Reiki, to which has been added four symbols of Tibetan origin, one of which is the equivalent of kundalini.

Transcendental Meditation (TM). An occult form of meditation derived from yoga and promoted in the West by Maharishi Mahesh Yogi. Through the continuous repetition of a Sanskrit mantra, the meaning of which is withheld from the practitioner, it aims at producing an altered state of consciousness. Though promoters claim it is non-religious, the puja initiation involves the invocation of Hindu gods and the mantra is commonly an invocation of a Hindu god.

uncarved block. A metaphorical description of a human being at birth in Taoist philosophy, in which it is believed that one is born with a personal supply of Wu Chi creating a state of original innocence, in contrast to the Christian concept of original sin. As time progresses, this supply of chi rapidly becomes depleted. The aim of tai chi and chi kung is to restore the practitioner to the state of the uncarved block which allows one infinite creative possibilities.

Upanishads. The final and fourth book of the Vedas which treats of philosophical questions. A common thread running through them is the identity of the human soul with Brahman and the essential unity of all things.

Vedantic philosophy. The most common of the various Hindu philosophies exported to the West with yoga. Based on the belief that the only true reality is Brahman and all else in the cosmos is illusion, it is both monistic and pantheistic.

Vedas. The four books of Hindu scriptures believed to be a revelation from Brahman itself.

Vishnu. One of a group of three personal gods ranking immediately below the supreme impersonal god Brahman. In order, these are Brahma, the Creator, Vishnu the Preserver and Shiva the Destroyer, of whom Kundalini is the consort.

Western Reiki. A modified form of the 'secular Reiki' which Usui developed towards the end of his life for non-Buddhist disciples in Japan, and subsequently was transported to the West in a modified form by Mrs Takata. While claimed by adherents to be non-religious, its Buddhist roots are obvious. Currently, as a result of research into the origins of Japanese Usui Reiki, there is a strong move in the West to incorporate more Buddhist spirituality into the practice of Reiki to give it more 'bite'.

Wu Chi (The Tao). The ultimate source of chi in its highest form existing in a state of utter stillness and complete emptiness – 'the Great Void'; the supreme divinity of Taoist philosophy and commonly referred to in Reiki circles as 'the Source'.

Yoga. A series of physical poses accompanied by mind-altering processes such as retarded breathing, repetition of a mantra, or highly refined methods of concentration (raja yoga), and resulting at advanced levels in a sense of one's own divinity and the exercise of certain occult powers (siddhis).

yogi. An adept of yoga.

Zen. A school of Buddhism which places great stress on forms of meditation which aim at creating a void in the mind.

Lightning Source UK Ltd.
Milton Keynes UK
UKOW04f0243060815

256434UK00002B/37/P